D0849299

The New Rules of
AGING
WELL

ALSO BY FRANK LIPMAN, MD, AND DANIELLE CLARO

The New Health Rules

The New Rules of
AGING
WELL

A Simple Program
for Immune Resilience,
Strength, and Vitality

Frank Lipman, MD, and Danielle Claro

Photographs by Gentl & Hyers

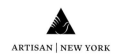

ARTISAN | NEW YORK

Library of Congress Cataloging-in-Publication Data

Names: Lipman, Frank, 1954– author. | Claro, Danielle, author.
Title: The new rules of aging well / Frank Lipman, MD, and Danielle Claro.
Description: New York : Artisan, a division of Workman Publishing Co., Inc. [2020]
Identifiers: LCCN 2020011410 | ISBN 9781579659592 (hardcover)
Subjects: LCSH: Older people—Health and hygiene. | Middle-aged people—Health and hygiene. | Self-care, Health. | Longevity
Classification: LCC RA777.6 .L5675 2020 | DDC 613/.0438—dc23
LC record available at https://lccn.loc.gov/2020011410

Design by Jane Treuhaft

Artisan books are available at special discounts when purchased in bulk for premiums and sales promotions as well as for fund-raising or educational use. Special editions or book excerpts also can be created to specification. For details, contact the Special Sales Director at the address below, or send an e-mail to specialmarkets@workman.com.

For speaking engagements, contact speakersbureau@workman.com.

Published by Artisan
A division of Workman Publishing Co., Inc.
225 Varick Street
New York, NY 10014-4381
artisanbooks.com

Artisan is a registered trademark of Workman Publishing Co., Inc.

Published simultaneously in Canada by Thomas Allen & Son, Limited

Printed in China

First printing, October 2020

10 9 8 7 6 5 4 3 2 1

With my lightning bolts a-glowing
I can see where I am going.

—*Arcade Fire*

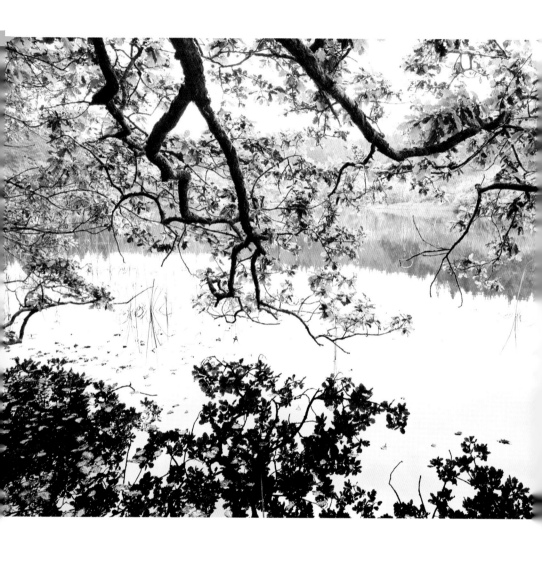

CONTENTS

PREFACE

In my medical practice, there's something I see again and again: patients in their 40s and 50s who feel as if they've been betrayed by their bodies. They're gaining weight, feeling exhausted, experiencing aches and pains, generally going south. They find that they're getting sick more often, catching everything they're exposed to and taking longer to recover.

People come to me assuming that these "symptoms of aging" are unavoidable. I tell them what I'm going to tell you now: These problems—losing mental sharpness, looking puffy, feeling generally lousy—are absolutely *not* a given of aging. They're a call to action, a sign that you need to change your lifestyle. When patients follow my advice—when they improve their lifestyle—the impact is often immediate.

I've had my own practice in New York City for more than 30 years, a blend of Chinese medicine and Western medicine. But even with my decades of experience, I personally had an awakening in my mid-50s. I changed a few things (habits I once believed were healthy choices), and quickly saw results. These days I'm often mistaken for someone decades younger.

Much of what's effective goes back to the principles of Chinese medicine. Older cultures get so much right about physiological processes and staying vital and strong decade after decade. Now cutting-edge research confirms this thinking. My advice on aging well and building immune resilience comes from this place: It's ancient wisdom backed up by modern science. And it's more important than ever. With new viruses appearing, it's critical to prioritize immunity and overall wellness. Aging does not have to make you more vulnerable. It can be a wake-up call to become the healthiest you've ever been.

There's no magic pill for health and immunity. There's a *lifestyle* that makes your immune system—and all other systems in the body—stronger. And I want to teach you that. That's why I joined forces with Danielle Claro to write this book—a straightforward guide that details the strategies I've seen work over and over again for patients in their 40s, 50s, 60s, and beyond. A blueprint for optimal function.

It contains everything I teach my patients, and then some, about turning around the so-called symptoms of aging— getting to your ideal weight, staying strong and nimble, sleeping well, enjoying life more—all of which plays into immune resilience. In many cases, this regimen has people looking and feeling younger at 60 than they did at 45.

The ordinary choices you make each day can have extraordinary effects on your overall health and your body's ability to protect itself. You only need to know what to do. I'm thrilled to say, the secrets you need are all right here.

—FRANK LIPMAN, MD

INTRODUCTION

You know that guy at work you thought was 50 and turned out to be 70? Or that woman in yoga class who seemed 40 until she introduced you to her 30-year-old kid? This book is here to help you become like them. To let you in on the health habits of people who age amazingly well—who look great, feel well, and are energetic, happy, sexy, agile, strong. It's not luck, and it's not something that's randomly bestowed on people. It's a result of specific life choices, and it's something anyone can have with motivation and commitment.

How you age has everything to do with the choices you make right now—what you eat and how active you are, but also how you spend your free time and how you see the world around you. There's a lot to it, and yet in some ways it's simple: What you put into your body and mind affects the whole organism, determining function and resilience.

If you're not aging well, there are answers: elements you need to add to your daily life (certain practices, foods, supplements) and others you need to subtract (same list, but different specs). Your body is a complex machine, and keeping it humming along beautifully as you age calls for a plan—one that preps your body to handle whatever the world throws at it.

Aging optimally is not just about living long. It's about being vital and happy and continuing to be able to do the things you love for decades to come. It means tuning in to your own health, becoming your own personal wellness coach, and learning to sense what you need when you need it. It involves responding to changes, preventing injury, building resilience, and being open to new approaches and new behaviors.

Reconsider what you've been told

In your 40s and 50s, your body begins naturally shifting into a mode where it's taking care of what's there—maintaining— because it's not producing and growing anymore; hormones shift, and cellular function is generally less efficient. But you can still thrive.

If you're achy, tired, gaining weight, not sleeping well, pay attention: These are warning signs. Signals from your body to get your sh*t together while you still can.

This is not a drill. If you want your body to run well as you age, you can't be cavalier anymore about how you treat it. Otherwise, what can happen is that your organs and other systems underperform; this is what makes you feel physically terrible from day to day and weakens your immunity over time. The right choices can radically alter, and even reverse, some of the symptoms our culture has come to accept as normal signs of aging.

You have power in this situation. Some folks worry that they're destined to age a certain way because of the way their relatives did. Nope. The idea of "bad genes" creating your destiny is grossly exaggerated. You can look at your family and gather useful information. You can get genome testing and learn a lot. But this info is only the beginning of the story, because lifestyle choices have a tremendous impact on whether certain genes turn on or off. Studies on identical twins prove this: How you age, in many ways, is up to you.

It's never too late to start

Don't despair or get stuck on changes you wish you'd made sooner. Many studies show that it's never too late to launch new habits and see results. Improvements make a difference at any age, and at any point in your health journey. Today is a great day to start. You'll notice positive effects pretty quickly.

Building a strong immune system

All the advice in this book—from when and how you eat to how much you sleep to what type of exercise you get—is designed to build immune resilience. Many of your immune cells turn over every month. How well they function is a direct response to the way you take care of yourself. Sure, there's some loss of function as we age, but it's a myth that weak immunity is a given after a certain point. We're going to show you the everyday practices and larger life philosophy that keep immunity hardy.

One of the most important things that happens when you're taking good care of yourself is that the immune system's self-cleaning mechanism, known as autophagy, kicks in on a daily basis. The definition of autophagy (accent on the second syllable—*au-TAHF-a-gee*) is digestion of cellular waste by enzymes of the same cell. In other words, it's your cells cleaning up their own debris. When your autophagy is bright and awake and working well, your body recovers faster and better. Everything in this book helps boost autophagy and keep the immune system operating optimally.

Nurturing your longevity genes

There are 20 or so genes that researchers have recently identified as "longevity genes"—those with the potential to help us live longer, healthier lives. Some you may have heard of are the sirtuins AMPK and mTOR.

The pathways of many of these longevity genes respond to lifestyle habits: what, when, and how much you eat; how you move your body; how much restful sleep you get; and how much stress you endure, among other things. Regulating these gene pathways up or down through healthy habits can extend your life span and expand your "health span"—the vitality level throughout your life—and that's what this book is all about.

Small "stresses" make you stronger

An overarching theme of nurturing your longevity genes and aging well is the concept of hormesis. Hormesis is your body's response to small healthy stresses—say, fasting for a short time, or biking up a brief, steep hill. These little stresses, or short periods of adversity, stimulate the body's defenses against aging without doing harm. You'll hear a lot about hormesis as we continue. It's an easy umbrella under which a lot of our advice lives, and it can help you think about self-maintenance in a new way. Small stresses regarding food, exercise, and temperature are challenges you're going to seek out from now on. It's a playful, proactive way to approach wellness, and a great way to reframe necessities like stepping outside on an ice-cold morning to walk the dog (skip the coat).

Cues from nature

Your body is smart. It has the ability and the inclination to link with larger natural cycles: day and night, the change of seasons. All your organs have rhythms. When you work *with* your body clock—eating, sleeping, and exercising when your body is most primed to do so—your systems can work efficiently. When you don't, your body is forced to compensate, which takes energy away from important processes. It's the difference between swimming with the current and fighting your way upstream. Throughout this book, we encourage you to take advantage of that current, to use what's already there, the natural built-in rhythms of healthy living. This makes it so much easier to age well.

Mitochondria and telomeres

Mitochondrial function and telomere length are aging mechanisms that come up throughout this book. Mitochondria, as you may know, are the energy powerhouses of the cells. Autophagy—the body's self-cleaning system, mentioned above—helps mitochondria stay strong, which in turn makes you feel and look better. Research is uncovering more every day about the significance of mitochondria to healthy aging.

Telomeres are the caps on the ends of DNA strands—like aglets on the tips of a shoelace. A recent Harvard study brought to light the importance of telomeres in our understanding and possible manipulation of the effects of aging. Long, strong telomeres indicate youth and health. Bad habits shorten telomeres. The lifestyle we teach in this book is designed to keep telomeres as long and strong as possible.

———

The science is important, but what it looks like in real life is simple everyday choices; that's what builds immune resilience and helps certain people age spectacularly. This book is here to teach the right habits and help you implement them. Once in place, these practices keep autophagy kicking in daily, make your mitochondria efficient, maintain the length and strength of telomeres, minimize inflammation, build immune resilience, and much more. When these systems are thriving, everything else works well too.

It's not always easy to make changes. But there's momentum to good habits. Locking in one makes the next one easier to add, and the one after that even more of a breeze. Pretty soon you don't even need to think about them. You're reflexively making great choices. You're supporting your body. You're optimizing function. All systems are go. You're aging well.

Stay with us. We're going to help you get to that place. You won't believe how great you're going to feel.

LEVEL 1:

THE ESSENTIALS

———

Powerful changes you can make today
to strengthen immunity, increase energy,
and age better immediately

Just. Eat. Less.

The biggest factor in healthy aging is simply eating less. After about age 45, your body just doesn't need as many calories as it once did—it's not building anymore; it's protecting and preserving. This requires less fuel.

A recent study showed that subjects who reduced calories by 30 percent lived longer and even avoided some age-related diseases. This research didn't even take into account what the subjects were eating, only the amount. So this single change—eating less now, and cutting back a little more every five years or so—can have a serious impact.

Consuming less food is also easier on your system. Less food means less for your body to process, less garbage for it to dispose of. It lightens the workload, and that translates into better overall function.

It may sound like a big ask. We get that. Some of the happiest times in life are centered around food. Time around the table with family and friends is precious and, in fact, also an important part of aging well—community, love, sharing, connection. Just be smart about what's *on* that table and be conscious of habits that need tweaking. Do you always overeat when you're with certain friends? With your family of origin? When you drink? When you're feeding others? Parenting can be very food-centric, but as kids get older, life becomes less about three meals a day; you may be at a place where you can tune in to your own needs (and adjust for age), rather than eat according to the clock.

Obviously, one of the most effective ways to reduce calories is to cut out starchy and refined carbs. Bread, pasta, rice, and other white foods (cauliflower notwithstanding) are not only basically devoid of nutrients but are also potentially dangerous. Most of us lose the ability to process carbs well as we age—that's why there's an increased risk of diabetes (carbs turn to sugar in the body). This is serious. More than 100 million adults in the United States have diabetes or prediabetes. Cutting empty carbs in favor of nutrient-dense foods is one important way to lower your risk. A note: When we talk about diabetes in this book, we're referring to type 2 diabetes, a condition caused by lifestyle habits, not type 1 diabetes, which is an autoimmune disease.

Of course, food can be complicated. At times, the perception of hunger may be a need for something else—distraction, affection, exercise, fresh air, sleep, even just water. Eating less is about staying alert, being sensitive to your body, and watching out for automatic behaviors (heading straight to the kitchen the minute you walk in the door, say, without stopping to wonder if you're actually even hungry).

Start with the simple idea of eating till you're only 80 percent full. It's the difference between satisfying your hunger and feeling the need to unbutton your pants. This alone can be life-altering.

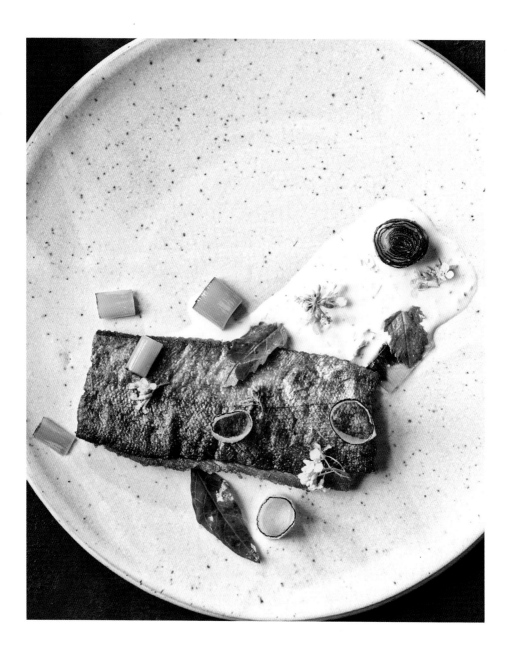

16-hour overnight fasting

Short fasts benefit you in a few ways. One is simple calorie reduction: When you don't eat for an extended period of time, you naturally (and effortlessly) eat less overall. Another is that your digestive system works better when it has a chance to rest and recover—and in fact, your body can repair itself better when it isn't constantly diverting energy to digestion. Third, fasting causes major changes in several crucial hormones that impact aging and weight, including insulin and growth hormone. Fourth, fasting is one of those hormetic "small stresses" that stimulate the longevity gene pathways. Fifth—and this is big—fasting kicks in autophagy, the cellular detox process critical to strong immunity and aging well.

So here's the plan: A couple of times a week, have dinner on the early side, and the first meal the next day a little later, leaving a good 16 hours in between. This simple practice is incredibly powerful. And it's not that difficult. You make it a point to finish dinner by 7 or 8 p.m. You're sleeping for seven or eight hours, we hope (see page 30). In the morning, you get up and have a big glass of water. And then you eat a nice nutritious meal at 11 or 12.

Admittedly, fasting can be a challenge at first. You don't have to go from zero to 16 if this sounds insane to you. Start with 12 hours, then move to 14, building to 16. Once your body adjusts, fasting feels great and is weirdly liberating. Realizing that you don't need to eat all the time—that your body functions well and doesn't require constant loading—is freeing, and helps you break that carb addiction. Soon you'll find your fasting days refreshing: less of a sacrifice and more of a break. And you may find that mornings are especially productive when you've taken food out of the equation.

Here are answers to some frequently asked questions about fasting.

What's the difference between 16-hour fasting, intermittent fasting, and time-restricted eating?

There isn't really a difference. They're just different ways of saying the same thing, which is that it's a good idea to have a window during which you eat (we suggest eight hours) and a longer stretch of time when that window is closed (we suggest 16 hours).

Why 16 hours?

Because studies show that it takes about 16 hours of fasting for autophagy to kick in and do its job. Feel free to do 18 or 20 hours if you like.

What if I can't go 16 hours?

Do what you can. Any short fast is a good fast. Twelve hours is better than 10, and 14 is better than 12. If you increase gradually, it may be easier than you think.

How often should I do this?

Start with two days a week. Generally, newbies find it easier to fast on workdays. The ultimate goal is to do this all the time, with 16 hours between your last meal of the day and your first meal the following day. Folks who do find it very comfortable and report weight loss, increased energy, and better sleep. If that feels unrealistic to you, don't sweat it. Get yourself up to three days a week, and you'll notice benefits.

But what about my midnight snack?

If you're a night snacker, you need to find ways to close down the food portion of your day. On fasting nights, clean up and shut down the kitchen right after dinner, so you have no need to step in there. If you're a morning eater who wakes up starving, the first couple of fasts can be a challenge. When your body adjusts, you won't wake up craving food. You're reprogramming yourself. It may take a little while, and improving your diet as you go will help.

What if I exercise in the morning?

It's actually great to exercise without eating because there's no glucose being used for energy, so your body burns fat. It's a myth that you have to eat something before you exercise.

Can I have water?

Yes, water is great in the morning because it rehydrates you and can get things moving.

Can I have coffee in the morning?

The jury's still out on whether it's okay to have coffee while fasting. Strictly speaking, the answer is no. Some folks (including us) go with the theory that a cup of coffee or tea with no carbs or protein does not end your fast. Others say that as soon as you have anything but water—including black coffee—the liver is working. We don't quite know yet. If it's easy for you to go 16 hours with nothing but water, go for it. That's ideal, and you'll probably feel amazing. If you do have coffee or tea, don't use regular milk or half-and-half (and definitely don't use sugary alternatives like sweetened almond or oat milk), because they contain carbs and protein, which will cause your body to secrete insulin. It's important not to trigger insulin, so if you need something in your coffee, use a pure fat like MCT (medium-chain triglycerides) oil, which contains no carbs or protein. To review: Best is just water. Second-best is tea or coffee without sugar or milk. Third is tea or coffee with MCT oil.

What about longer fasts?

There's not just one way to do this. Intermittent fasting is pretty easy, and there are a few variations you might want to look into. But if you want to explore more intensive fasting—like one whole day per week with no food, or multiple days of water-fasting—don't do it without the supervision of your doctor.

What about the fasting-mimicking diet I keep hearing about?

Researcher Valter Longo's fasting-mimicking diet shows excellent results. It's a good option if you prefer it. For five consecutive days once a month, you eat very little—a low-calorie, low-carb, low-protein diet (no animal protein); it has positive effects on aging biomarkers. This diet lines up completely with the rest of the advice in this book. You can go to ProLonFMD .com to learn more.

What if fasting doesn't get easier for me?

If your diet contains a lot of sugar and starch, fasting can be harder in the beginning. Take a week to cut way back on sugar, drop all grains, and even eliminate legumes. Then try again, and see if fasting is a bit easier. It should be.

Is 16-hour fasting safe for everyone?

There are some people who shouldn't fast. Don't fast if you're on multiple medications, if you're an athlete training at a high level, if you're extremely stressed, or if you have a history of disordered eating. Although fasting stresses the system in a good way, it could be too much if your system is already overloaded from outside stressors. If you're in a rough place emotionally, fasting may not be the best move for you. Obviously, if you're pregnant, don't fast. Kids shouldn't fast. If you have any concerns, check with your doctor first.

The gut–immunity connection

Seventy percent of the immune system is found in the gut. As you age, it's critical to cultivate a healthy gut microbiome, full of many different strains of good bacteria (and low on bad bacteria). If that internal ecosystem is off, it makes your delicate gut wall vulnerable (among other things), which can lead to serious issues throughout your body.

Your gut wall is the primary barrier between your body and the outside world (where food, bugs, toxins can be threats). Protecting that barrier—which determines what's allowed into your system and what's not—is the key to health.

When the microbiome is not healthy and balanced, your fragile woven gut wall loosens, leaving tiny spaces where bacteria, toxins, and pieces of partially digested food can leak into the bloodstream. This is called "leaky gut," and it's as bad as it sounds. The particles can set off inflammation almost anywhere in your system. This is all internal, but the effects are not subtle. Leaky gut can trigger joint pain, skin rashes, moodiness, anxiety, depression, brain fog, and hormonal issues. It can weaken immunity and exacerbate autoimmune problems. Many of the issues we chalk up to aging could in fact be the result of an imbalanced microbiome—which you can do something about.

It begins with your diet. But there's more. Almost all the advice in this book contributes to the strength and wellness of the gut microbiome. The short version is: Eat fresh, organic, unprocessed food; stay away from antibiotic-treated and hormone-riddled animal products—and produce that's been sprayed with toxic herbicides like glyphosate (certified organic growers do not spray with glyphosate). Feed your body prebiotics (garlic, onions, leeks, asparagus) and probiotics (fermented foods) every day. Sleep, hydrate, meditate, use antibiotics only when you absolutely need them, and don't take stomach medications like Nexium for long periods. In other words, many of the lifestyle habits that are good for general wellness are also key for gut health and immunity as you age. And everything you need to help your gut thrive is right here in this book.

Get serious about cutting sugar

Sugar is extra harmful as you age. It weakens the immune system and feeds diseases we all fear: diabetes, heart disease, cancer, and Alzheimer's, to name a few.

In combination with certain proteins, sugar creates deposits that get into the bloodstream. They become lodged in various places and sit like rust on your organs (on the skin, which is your largest organ, this manifests as wrinkles). These deposits also damage cell membranes and can bore tiny holes in the walls of blood vessels. If you make only one change, it should be cutting refined sugar from your diet (and honey and agave too—it's essentially all the same to your system). Sugar is hiding in a lot of processed foods, but start with the obvious stuff: cereal, cookies, candy, soda, fruit juice (which, incidentally, is just as bad for you as soda). Delete, delete, delete.

When you really need something sweet, eat some berries or a green apple (lower in sugar than most apples). The fiber in fruit slows the absorption of sugar somewhat, which minimizes the sudden rush and subsequent plummet of your blood sugar caused by standard sweets.

A little sugar in your coffee adds up to a lot over time; wean yourself off. But don't use artificial sweeteners, which are full of chemicals. If you really want to sweeten your coffee or tea, try monk fruit—which looks like table sugar, and also comes in drops—or Stevia; get pure Stevia, because some Stevia products contain other sweeteners. To be honest, neither really tastes like sugar, but they are sweet. Use them to transition away from a sweet tooth, because the goal is to retrain your palate to stop craving sugar. Some folks opt for sugar alcohols such as erythritol and xylitol, but they can give you gas and upset your digestion, so better to avoid them.

Even though our culture frames sugar as a treat—dessert is an indulgence, sometimes a reward—it's actually more like a punishment for your body. And it's so hard to break away from because it's a drug, an addictive substance that stimulates the same areas in the brain as cocaine and heroin. You should be afraid of it.

If you're really sugar-dependent and struggling to cut back, the supplement glutamine could be helpful. It basically tricks the brain into thinking you're getting glucose. You might want to try taking it during your first few weeks tapering off sugar.

Sleep more and sleep better

One of the goals of this book is to help you improve your life *before* aches and pains arrive. Daily recovery—high-quality sleep—is a critical piece of this puzzle as you age. Prioritize sleep, and you'll feel better right away.

Much of what people think of as signs of aging are just signs that the body needs more (and better) regular rest. If falling asleep or staying asleep has become a challenge, don't give up. Instead, pay attention to the problem and consciously set yourself up for a good night's sleep. This is not just about how you orchestrate your evening; it's also about daytime habits. Step outside into the sunshine first thing in the morning to keep your circadian rhythms in sync with nature (lively in the day, waning as the sun sets, sleepy at night). Meditate in the morning; this has a positive impact on p.m. sleep—as does exercise: Cardio workouts during the day make it easier to fall asleep at night.

It's important to get enough REM sleep—when dreaming happens—and also deep sleep, which is a type of non-REM

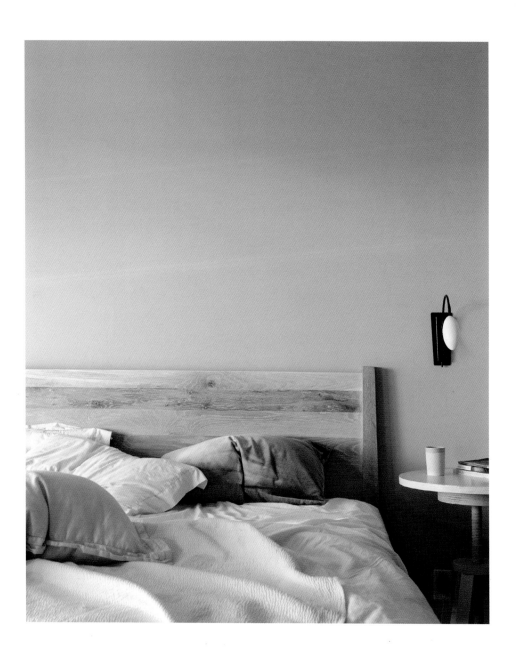

sleep when there's very little brain activity. This is when recovery is happening in the body, and when the brain's cleansing system (known as the glymphatic system) kicks in to clear protein and other toxins. If you don't sleep well and miss out on deep sleep, the glymphatic system is not able to do its job. As a result, all this stuff builds up in the brain, leaving you feeling foggy and off.

Most people do best with seven to nine hours of sleep. Yes, nine. If TV, social media, or endless work emails are stealing away your sleep hours, change that.

Sleep interruptions are not necessarily a given of aging. Yes, there are times when hormones will mess with you and interfere with falling or staying asleep. And as you get older, you'll probably need to get up to pee more often in the night. If you make some extra effort, you should be able to get back to sleep pretty easily. Before you throw your hands up and say, "I just don't sleep well anymore," check these factors.

That 3 p.m. latte. How you metabolize caffeine is a genetic thing (genome testing like 23andMe can test for this, in fact). Some people can have caffeine after dinner and conk out at bedtime; others are so sensitive, they feel jittery all day from one cup of morning coffee. Caffeine can have a half-life of seven hours, meaning that seven hours after you drink a cup of coffee, half the caffeine is still in your body. Know your limits. If you're sensitive to caffeine, cut it off at 2 p.m., latest.

Wine with dinner. Alcohol disrupts the sleep cycle, so even if you think it helps you wind down, it can wake you up in the night. Also, wine and beer are high in carbs and turn to sugar in the body.

Light creeping in. Light interferes with your body's production of melatonin, a natural sleep hormone. Make your bedroom totally dark, and cover charging lights with black tape. When you get up to use the bathroom, don't turn on a bright light or check your phone.

An overheated bedroom. You need a lower core body temperature for sleep; being too warm could inhibit sleep hormones. A hot bath an hour or so before bed actually *lowers* your core temperature, which is good. There are also cooling mattress toppers that might make a difference. Keep the thermostat low or the windows open.

A bedtime snack. Late-night eating wakes up your digestive system and, if you consume carbs, can bring on a sugar rush. There are lots of other reasons not to eat at night, including the fact that it contributes to weight gain (see page 195).

Falling asleep in front of the TV. The blue light of the screen inhibits melatonin production. Same thing with reading on an iPad or looking at a laptop. That blue light is telling your body to stay awake. Then, of course, there's the brain stimulation from the show you're watching, and micro-arousals from the audio once you nod off. All these factors interfere with sleep. If you just use the TV as background noise to help you get out of your head, try a sound machine instead.

Lots of everyday physical activity

Exercise as you age is not just about defined workouts. It's about moving as much as you can every single day, all day long, in regular daily life. Be a physical person. An active life overall is more beneficial than an hour at the gym (especially if that hour comes between a day at a desk and a night on the couch). Of course, gym time is also great. But the real key to aging well is to be active every chance you get.

Besides keeping the body and mind vital and sharp, physical activity fends off stress and depression, improves circulation, promotes higher-quality sleep, builds immune resilience, and reduces the risk of chronic diseases.

As you age, it's important to take extra care with exercise— it should be less about heavy exertion and more about frequency. Don't take this the wrong way, but your body is breaking down. All our bodies are. After 40 or so (or even the late 30s), muscles shift from a state of growth to one of preservation. The focus at this point? Conserving, maintaining, and, most important, preventing injury. The mantra is "do no harm," because as you get older, your capacity to heal lessens.

Your body is always busy maintaining health, constantly repairing (from everyday wear and tear), dealing with germs and toxins (in our world and in our food), working hard to keep things right. When you, say, sprain an ankle, some of the energy that goes to daily maintenance has to be diverted. Your body needs to produce enzymes and anti-inflammatory nutrients to repair that ankle, and this may detract from its ability to keep up with other necessary recovery. Because resources decrease as we age, it's smart to be protective. Not getting injured is a positive, proactive thing you can do to maintain overall health. Of course, injuries can also indirectly age you, since low-grade inflammation is one of the causes of aging more rapidly.

The key is to adapt your fitness routine as your body changes, be open to gentler workouts, and if something hurts, *don't do it*. Sounds obvious, but a lot of us ignore pain and push through. That mentality is not great for aging well. It's much better to adjust, pull back, change it up. If you discover that you can't run pain-free anymore, ride a bike. If you can't ride, swim. If it hurts to jump into a yoga push-up, step back instead. This can be tough, because a lot of us are attached to our activities and consider them essential to our identity. But it's more important to preserve than to push. If you were an Iron Man in your 30s, you've got to acknowledge that it may not be appropriate for you in your 50s. You need your muscles and joints forever, so think twice before wearing them out. Being nimble at 90 depends on how you take care of yourself now. For those of you who love to move and to push yourselves physically, the most important thing is to adapt as the body tells you to.

For those folks who are not active, the directive is to start exercising now. It's never too late. Walk a slight hill for 10 minutes a day to begin. Extend that by five minutes each week till you're up to 30 minutes a day. Restorative yoga is another great entry point, as are aqua classes, which are light on joints. Ease in and build consistently. It doesn't take long—or take much—to transform yourself into an active person.

And for all of us: Welcome opportunities to move, all day long. Take an earlier train so you can get off a stop or two sooner and walk to the office, or get off the bus early to add some footwork to your trip home. Skip the elevator for the stairs on the way up (not the way down—going down stairs or hills can be tough on the knees). Make your lunch break a movement break (and when possible, an outdoor fresh-air break). It's not necessarily about exerting yourself a lot; it's about constant, consistent, dependable activity. Be a mover.

Watch the alcohol and other toxins

As you age, your capacity to break down alcohol decreases. You may have noticed this if you've found yourself tossing and turning in bed after a second glass of wine with dinner. You used to be fine having two glasses, and now you're not. That's a normal consequence of aging, and one you can address. Alcohol is not good for your body for a few reasons (among them, it weakens the immune system and ups your sugar intake), but the fact that it interferes with sleep is especially problematic, because of the domino effect: If you're not rested, your body craves sugar and carbs (for quick energy); you might be too tired to exercise; you overdo it on caffeine and throw off your internal clock, which messes up your next night's sleep. Not to mention feeling crummy and being snappish. One bad night leads to another, and you become more exhausted (and more prone to reach for carbs), and the cycle continues. Isn't it easier just to skip that second glass?

Also, be real about alcohol. The polyphenols—antioxidants found in some flavonoid-rich foods like grape skins, blueberries, cocoa, and tea—in dry red wine have boosted its cred as a good choice, and compared to other forms of alcohol, it is. It's *better*. But it's not like it's good for you. If it's polyphenols you're after, get them from high-quality black or green tea. Wine is not the best delivery system.

People ask about tequila: 100 percent agave tequila is low in sugar, but it's usually served with a sugary mixer. Straight up, it's low in carbs, as is vodka with seltzer (not tonic, which is very high in sugar).

Look, alcohol is a toxin, but context matters. Sharing a drink with friends or family can be nourishing in an emotional way. So we're not saying never. If you have a glass of wine a couple of times a week and it's not having negative effects, it's not a problem. But you shouldn't be drinking every day. And obviously, if you *have* to have alcohol, that's an issue, and something to deal with.

Four big glasses of water a day

As you age, the thirst signal can fade. This is not the case for everyone, but some people just don't get the memo; although the body wants water, it doesn't convey that to the mouth as clearly as it once did. Lack of fluids might express itself in other ways: loss of energy, irritability, fuzziness. So any feeling you have, start with water: if you can't concentrate, if your partner's voice is irking you, if you feel unable to cope, if you have a headache. Water it. Brain function can be affected by dehydration. Every day, drink at least four big glasses of water—ideally filtered water; the chlorine in tap water can attack the good bacteria in your microbiome, and a filter can minimize that problem. Find smart options for water filters at EWG.org, the site for the Environmental Working Group.

Hydration is more effective if you drink over the course of the day rather than stand by the sink guzzling your allotment. Drink anytime, with meals or without—it all counts. If you don't love water, infuse it with a handful of mint leaves or a squeeze of citrus. Make a pitcher or fill a large ball jar and leave it in the fridge. Lemon in water stimulates liver function. Wash citrus rind or cucumber skin if you're dropping unpeeled produce into your water.

Tea counts toward hydration, by the way, but coffee doesn't (it's a diuretic). Seltzer made from filtered water (SodaStream at home, say) is fine. Regular seltzer may not be made with filtered water, so that's not great. Don't drink flavored seltzers; chemicals are used to achieve those "natural" flavors. We're not against bubbles, per se. The important part is where the water comes from, and what's been added to it.

We assume that it goes without saying, but don't drink soda or juice (fructose is as problematic as the sugar in soda), and no energy drinks, please. Also no bottled iced tea, which is full of chemicals and artificial sweeteners. Pretty much anything in a bottle at a deli besides water is problematic in one way or another. Cutting out bottled drinks is an easy way to lower your intake of sugar and chemicals. Just. Drink. Water.

Grow your tribe

Cultivating connection and spending time with people you love is a huge factor in aging well. In certain phases of life, there's no shortage of community: We have a built-in tribe at school and then at work; for parents, there's community involved in raising kids. But as circumstances change—you switch jobs, the kids go off to college, you retire—you might need to make some effort. And this effort—seeing friends, tending important relationships, cultivating new connections—is very important to your health. Don't wait for life transitions; prioritize socializing right now.

Think how good it feels to sit with a friend and talk and laugh. That should be the rule, not the exception. Make it happen one way or another at least weekly. Consider socializing a wellness activity, and figure out what you can change in order to weave in more time with dear friends.

As for making new friends—obviously, it's tricky as an adult. It's easy to say, "Find people who like to do what you like to do," but it takes time. So think of this as an invitation into a fresh mindset—one of planting seeds and seeing what comes up. Be alert and aware when you meet folks you like. Notice, observe, and open up to the notion of hanging out with new people. Let your interests lead you, and you'll gradually end up finding kindred spirits. At this point in your life, isolation might not be a risk, but one of the reasons to build a strong loving social structure around yourself now is to ensure that it doesn't become an issue later. You want to have plenty going on so there's cushioning all around when life transitions hit.

As you get older, you need to have a tribe, a real community, people who will listen to you, who will pick you up—emotionally and literally (say, when you need a ride home after a dental procedure). We're wired to need some type of family. Without that, studies show incontrovertibly that we age quicker. And with it, specifically with plenty of social contact in middle age and later in life, the risk of dementia drops.

In the "blue zones"—those places around the world where people live longest and are healthy beyond our wildest imaginings—there are three things you see across the board: lots of movement in daily life, a sense of purpose, and communal living. Build and cultivate your community. Have people over. Say yes to invitations. Put in the time. It's more important than you think.

Have a sense of humor about aging

Your attitude has a big impact on your health. Aging well involves cutting back on some classic pleasures—sweets, alcohol, fries, food in general—but if you can find a way to cultivate a positive approach, and stay cheerful about changes, it's much easier. Try to view dietary sacrifices as an opportunity to figure out what else you like and develop an appetite for learning or nature or meditation.

Be generous with yourself in other ways. What is it that feels good, brings excitement, and motivates you and also does no harm? Is it more time with certain friends? A class you've been wanting to take? An instrument you used to play?

Enjoy small healthy pleasures—a hot bath, a walk at sunset, a weekly treatment like an infrared sauna or massage. As you move into a place where you're making great choices, redefine the concept of indulgence and pepper your life with supportive, health-affirming practices.

You'll appreciate life more if you can stay light and positive. Embrace the changes, nurture your body and mind, and smile at the more humbling aspects that come with piling up the years. It's all a gift and, as they say, better than the alternative. Go with the flow, and you'll likely age better.

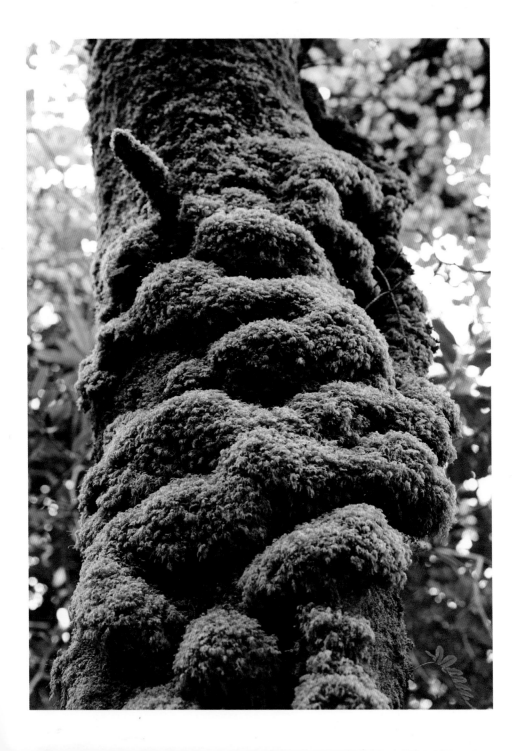

What a difference a fast makes

"**Will, 45,** has been married for five years and is the father of two little kids. He works for a tech start-up. He should be enjoying his family, but he feels like an old man. He's achy, tired, and depressed. He tells me it's exhausting for him to even sit and read to the kids. He feels like life is slipping away.

Will is 50 pounds overweight and on six different drugs that his last doctor prescribed: antihypertensives for his high blood pressure, Nexium for heartburn, diabetes medication, antidepressants, and Lipitor for his cholesterol. He takes Advil most nights for headaches. His inflammatory markers are high.

His office is full of salty and sweet snacks. There's free lunch every day. No one leaves the building for a break—it's frowned upon, because the work culture is so intense. The long hours wear him out, and his only breaks from his computer screen involve getting up to grab snacks, which he relies on to get him through the day. He says he's always munching on something and he never sees the sun.

I put Will on a low-carb diet, with intermittent fasting. We start with two days a week of 12-hour overnight fasts. He struggles with morning cravings for the first week but soon adjusts. Over the course of a month, I have Will increase to four days a week of 16-hour fasts. Will gets into it. Fasting helps him get out the door faster in the mornings, and creates some much-needed parameters around food. He finds that he's less hungry in general. And when he starts dropping weight, he's even more motivated.

He drinks more water and green tea, and finds that after a few weeks of eating a low-carb diet and fasting for 16-hour periods, his cravings for snacks decrease. At lunchtime, Will takes a brisk walk around the block to get some sunshine and exercise before eating. He makes better picks at the cafeteria buffet, where there are plenty of fresh vegetables to choose from.

Will slowly tapers off his Nexium. At night if he feels a headache coming on, he drinks water, and this helps. The headaches become less frequent, and when Will does experience one, he takes a little CBD oil for relief—no more Advil.

After a month, he's lost 20 pounds and his blood pressure is down to normal levels, so I start tapering him off the antihypertensive meds. His blood sugar drops significantly, and after two months, he doesn't need his diabetes meds anymore.

Will begins to make use of the good parts of his work environment—free group meditation in the morning, a few minutes of Ping-Pong to clear his head instead of a candy bar. When I see Will after three months, he's lost 40 pounds, his blood pressure remains normal without medication, and he no longer has diabetes. His inflammatory markers have normalized, and his cholesterol numbers have improved significantly. His energy is up. He no longer feels depressed, and he starts tapering off the antidepressants under my supervision. He's telling funny stories about his kids, bubbling over with enthusiasm, and says he feels 20 years younger. He has his life back. And after six months, he stops his Lipitor."

THINK ABOUT IT:

- How many meds are you on?

- Have you discussed with your doctor what those meds are doing for you, and if there's a lifestyle change that would allow you to stop taking them?

- What are the everyday "environmental factors" in your work world that are harming you? Stresses, snacks, schedules?

- Are there healthy things you can do for yourself in the midst of a busy day? What's available to you that you're not using?

- Have you tried intermittent fasting? If not, what's causing you to hesitate?

LEVEL 2:

EASY ADDS

––––––––––––––

Not every change geared toward
aging well is complex or difficult.
Here are a handful of simple tweaks
that can have profound effects.

Microbursts of physical intensity

Earlier, we talked about the concept of hormesis: the idea that low doses of acute physical stress produce a positive biological response. One way to spark hormesis and stimulate your longevity gene pathways is to pepper moderate workouts with short bursts of serious effort.

Whether you're walking uphill, biking, rowing, or swimming, you can inject regular intense microbursts into the session. How intense? Well, one measure of moderate exercise is that you're able to talk while doing it—your breathing comes easily enough that you could carry on a conversation. So during microbursts, you should be working so hard (and breathing so hard) that you can't chat.

Working out with a pattern that builds to microbursts is sometimes called high-intensity interval training (HIIT). It sounds specific, but it's nothing you can't craft on your own. A simple format you can apply to pretty much any type of exercise: Ramp up for 1 minute; go hard for 1 minute; drop back down to a comfortable pace for 3 minutes; repeat.

If you're just introducing the HIIT concept, do three rounds with this pattern, within an otherwise normal workout. As you become more comfortable, you can add more high-intensity intervals throughout the session. It can be fun and distracting, turning a monotonous activity (like swimming laps) into a bit of a game—and it's great for your body.

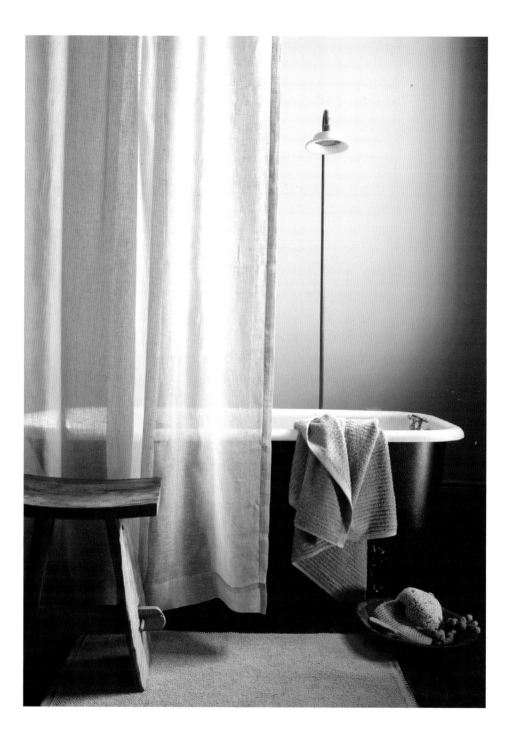

A cold rinse after a hot shower

▪▪▪▪▪▪▪▪▪▪▪▪▪▪▪▪▪▪▪▪

Real life provides many opportunities for hormesis—moments of "that which does not kill me makes me stronger." One of the easiest examples of this, and one of our favorites, is ending hot showers with 30 to 60 seconds of cold water.

On a gut level, you can just feel that this is good for you—it's instantly invigorating. It gets your chi (aka energy) flowing. And now in Western medicine, it's also on the books as a healthy practice. Research shows that it ups the production and health of your mitochondria.

Mitochondria are the energy sources of your cells—the essential force of life and longevity. They transform food and oxygen into ATP, or adenosine triphosphate, a type of molecule that powers biochemical reactions. ATP molecules are especially abundant in the cells of your heart, brain, and muscles. The advice in this book, on food, sleep, and nearly everything else, supports mitochondrial production and optimal function. And this little trick—a cold shower at the end of your hot one—does too.

The hot-to-cold principle works in reverse as well. Swim in a cool pool, then bask in a hot tub. Go back and forth between a sauna and a cold shower. Or just step outside in winter for a few minutes without a coat. It's so refreshing, especially after hours in an overheated indoor environment. That bracing shot of cold air is good for your body (in spite of what you may have been told as a kid).

The same principle of hormesis applies to other light stresses on the body, like short periods of fasting or bursts of challenging physical activity. These small challenges encourage autophagy, the body's cleaning system, and improve cellular function and repair.

As you get older, cellular function and the ability to repair diminish. The body can better repair damage when you give it these small acute stresses. "Damage" doesn't need to be anything dramatic. It's just the natural wear and tear of living and aging. Your body is always working to repair itself, and hormesis helps.

Rolling out the fascia

Very often it's not the muscle, it's the tight, constricted fascia that's causing pain in your body. Fascia is the stuff that encases the muscles, like a layer of Saran Wrap (think about that film on a raw chicken breast). As you age, it tightens. Stretching doesn't really get to tight fascia. It needs pressure to help it release, like what you'd get from a deep-tissue massage or from using a foam roller. Tight fascia doesn't just cause aches in muscles and joints; it can also change your gait and compromise your posture, generally making you look and feel old.

The solution is rolling out muscles regularly: Foam-rolling is as important to the body as exercise. You should be rolling out your muscles—quads, glutes, calves, deltoids, pectorals—a few times a week; it doesn't take long—just five or 10 minutes. This will help with existing pain and will also set you up better going forward. Rolling loosens the fascia and helps muscles work better, so it can prevent all sorts of injuries (as you age, you're more prone to injury). Because it makes your body mechanics more efficient, rolling can be your first line of defense against commonly recommended surgeries like hip or knee replacement.

At first, it may be a little painful in a "hurts so good" sort of way, but soon you'll become hooked on the relief you feel and how much better your body works. It's easier to follow a video than it is to read about how to foam-roll. Trainer Lauren Roxburgh has great step-by-step YouTube content. Pretty much any roller will do, so don't get overwhelmed by the available options. If you have a roller in the closet, pull it out and get started. The sensation is a little less intense if you set yourself up on a rug or an exercise mat.

Leave your roller in the living room or wherever you watch TV or otherwise hang out. Try a prompt, like whenever you're tempted to check social media, you roll out a body part first (customize this, so it works for you)—a.m., p.m., before and after exercise, while you talk on the phone.

Make rolling a habit. The more you do it, the better your body will feel.

Magnesium

––––––––––––

The mineral magnesium is one of the key nutrients for aging well; it's responsible for the correct metabolic function of more than 300 enzymes in the body. It supports the immune system, brings down blood pressure, aids brain and heart function, and helps you relax and fall asleep naturally. Quality sleep is like gold for longevity.

Spinach, pumpkin seeds, black beans, and wild-caught Pacific halibut are especially high in magnesium. But even with a good diet, 80 percent of us are deficient. So take a supplement.

There are a few different types, and it doesn't really matter which you choose. All varieties calm the nervous system, so it's great to take before bed, and you don't need to accompany it with food. Take 300 to 500 milligrams of magnesium glycinate or magnesium threonate. If you tend to be constipated, instead take magnesium citrate (400 to 600 milligrams) at night—it usually helps get things going by morning. If that dosage doesn't help with the constipation, increase slowly, up to 1,000 milligrams a night; decrease when you don't need as much. Buy the best-quality supplements you can afford. Good brands include Allergy Research Group, Pure Encapsulations, Thorne, The Well, and Designs for Health.

Magnesium can also be absorbed through the skin, in a bath. Ordinary Epsom salts are a form of magnesium, and a hot soak with them, as you probably know, is very soothing for overworked or tense muscles.

If you're curious about whether you're magnesium-deficient, ask your doctor to test your RBC magnesium (this is not the type most doctors check). You want that metric to fall between 5 and 6.5 milligrams per dL.

Sauna sessions

Preventing injury, supporting the immune system, curtailing illness, decreasing inflammation, improving circulation and heart health—these are central principles of aging well, and they're also benefits of sweating it out in a sauna. We're particularly fans of infrared saunas, because they're more comfortable than traditional saunas, which means you can stay in there and enjoy the effects for longer. An infrared sauna directly penetrates and heats the body rather than just heating the air around you. So it doesn't feel as extreme.

The infrared experience itself, for those who haven't tried it, is pretty straightforward. You're generally in a small-ish booth, and the heat can be adjusted to your preference (traditional saunas are typically heated to between 150°F and 180°F; infrared saunas work well at 120°F to 140°F). Often the lighting options offer a bit of color therapy (red is stimulating, blue is calming, and so on). There can be music. Even if you crank up the temperature, there's never that kind of oven-blast heat you get in a traditional sauna. It's eerily comfortable. You sweat a lot, which feels great, and afterward, you're quite energized. Sessions generally last 30 minutes.

It's harder to stay in a traditional sauna for that long, for sure, and we're not suggesting you do. Both types of saunas are great, and both can leave you feeling bright and lively, as long as you rehydrate. Drink, drink, drink after taking a sauna. Plain water is fine, but electrolyte-rich water like Catalyte by Thorne or Electrolyte Synergy by Designs for Health is even better; it helps replenish minerals lost through sweat.

Making saunas part of your life is a little like prioritizing sleep. It's an easy, gentle treat that also happens to be one of the best things you can do for your body—and a great go-to when you're not feeling well. If you sense a cold coming on, go for a sauna. Raising the body's core temperature stimulates your production of white blood cells, which fight off bacteria and viruses. It basically prompts your body's natural defense system to kick in quickly and powerfully. Saunas are also super helpful for achy muscles; for pain from inflammation, including arthritis; and for stress—a much better option than soothing yourself with carbs, sugar, or alcohol.

The cost of an infrared sauna session is not much more than you'd spend going out for a drink with a friend. Why not go together for a sauna and then take a walk instead? These replacement habits—new healthy indulgences—can gradually crowd out less-nourishing habits and will become your go-tos once you feel (and enjoy) the collective effects.

Medicinal mushrooms

Remember when we all upped our consumption of kale? It's time to do that with mushrooms. Current research shows that certain medicinal mushrooms—especially the varieties reishi, lion's mane, and chaga—contain high quantities of the antioxidants ergothioneine and glutathione, compounds known to prime the immune system and to help prevent the onset of Alzheimer's and Parkinson's. Lion's mane in particular is known as a "nootropic," which means it can enhance memory and cognitive function.

You can get these medicinal mushrooms via various delivery systems—powder, capsule, tincture—all of which seem to be effective. A nice place to start is with mushroom tea, which you can brew from a powder and drink on its own, or mix into bone broth, a smoothie, coffee, or black or green tea.

As tea, mushroom powders taste a bit earthy; some are a little bitter (those high in reishi) and some are subtle (chaga has vanilla undertones, and is delicious by itself). Have a couple of mugs a day. An organic powder we like is Four Sigmatic's 10 Mushroom Blend. If you prefer capsules, there's Host Defense's MyCommunity, a blend of 17 medicinal mushrooms. Both are available online.

These blends are extra powerful because they bring together the benefits of so many different kinds of medicinal mushrooms. If we had to choose only one mushroom for longevity and anti-aging, it would be reishi. It supports the immune system and cardiovascular health; it can lower blood pressure, reduce stress and inflammation, and even help prevent cancer. The mushroom lion's mane supports memory, cognitive function, and the nervous system. The combo products we recommend contain both reishi and lion's mane.

Integrating fresh organic mushrooms into your cooking or your salads is also beneficial—varieties like shiitake, maitake, and oyster all have medicinal and health-boosting properties.

For detailed info on the healing power of various types of mushrooms (and a lot more), there's a great book called *The Rebel's Apothecary: A Practical Guide to the Healing Magic of Cannabis, CBD, and Mushrooms*, by wellness expert Jenny Sansouci.

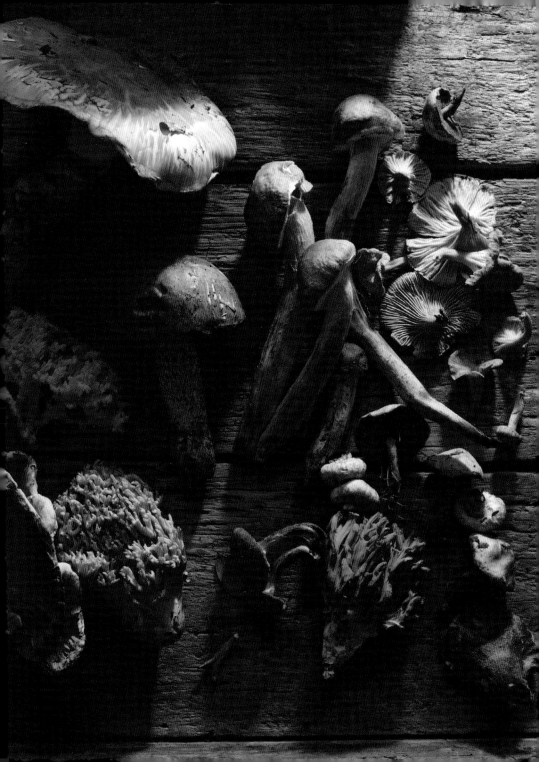

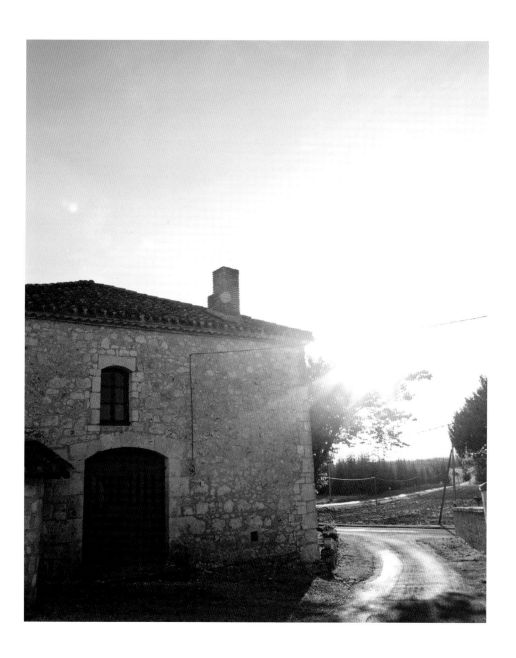

Sunshine in the morning

––––––––––––––––––

Circadian rhythms—or feeling the arc of a 24-hour day in conjunction with nature—are helpful in self-care. And sunshine, which we've been programmed to fend off with potentially toxic sunscreen, is good for your health. You don't want to always be covered up against sunlight. Get outside and feel the sun on your face and (season permitting) arms and legs every day.

One of the keys to feeling sleepy at night is to kick off your day with natural light. If you're lucky enough to have morning sun in your bedroom, let it stream in. Otherwise, get outside first thing, even for just a few minutes. This tells your body it's time to wake up, stops the flow of the sleep hormone melatonin, and sets up your internal clock to keep you energized during the day and help you wind down at night.

The timing of meals also has a powerful effect on your body clock. In terms of metabolic rhythm, your biggest meal should be at midday. If you eat late at night, your body thinks it's daytime (the time it needs calories and energy). This can negatively affect the secretion of sleep hormones, and that translates into trouble falling asleep, or a generally restless night. Without high-quality sleep, your body and brain miss out on essential self-cleaning and restoration. And then you're in that vicious cycle we mentioned earlier (you wake up unrested, you reach for carbs for energy, you have a late-afternoon coffee to stay alert, you find that you can't fall asleep that night, and so on). Taking your sleep life seriously is one of the most important things you can do for your health. Linking to daylight and darkness, connecting with nature in this very basic way, will help.

A bedtime ritual

Sleep and wake cycles are critical to wellness as you age. It's not just about quantity; it's also about quality: Your body and brain need a full complement of REM and non-REM sleep; deep sleep is part of the non-REM cycle. Going to bed at around the same time most nights and waking up around the same time most mornings helps lock in restorative sleep patterns. It's okay to sleep a bit later on weekends, but the concept of "catching up" on sleep is not a real thing. Your body needs *regular* daily recovery. If you're getting five hours a night during the week and sleeping till 11 a.m. on Sunday, that's going to be a problem.

A bedtime ritual can help. Like children, we do well with routines—they cue the body and mind to shift gears. It's helpful to have an official plan for tuning out the day, shaking away tense thoughts, and relaxing the body.

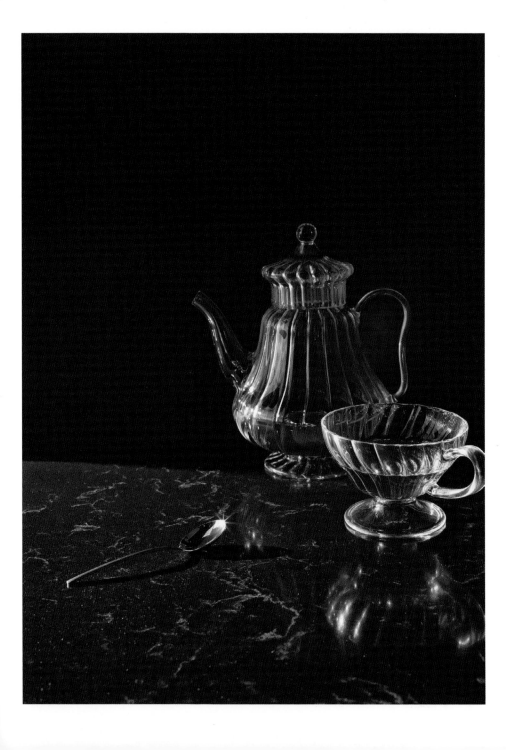

Rather than watching TV and eventually dragging your exhausted bones off to bed, make space for the transition. Start getting ready for bed an hour earlier than usual, and use the time to set yourself up for high-quality, truly restorative rest. Your bedtime ritual should take a little while—it's not something to rush through. This is time devoted to easing out of one state into another. Put together a routine that feels right. Pick from the ideas here or devise your own plan.

- Dim the lights an hour or two before you turn in.

- Relax your muscles with an Epsom salt soak. Add a couple of drops of soothing lavender oil.

- Relax your brain by dumping out whatever is in there: Make a to-do list or write in a journal. Pour out resentments or anger, and follow that exercise with a gratitude list.

- Think about what kind of content you consume at night. Some people can read a tense thriller and conk out, and others need to neutralize. A crossword puzzle, a YA novel (yes, adults can read these too), gentle poetry, spiritual essays. Find what works for you.

- If you can't turn off your brain, listen to relaxing music or use a white-noise machine.

It might seem like meditation is a fit here, but many people find meditating energizing. So we don't usually recommend meditating before bed. Breathwork can be nice, though, just concentrating on long, easy breaths: Inhale for a slow count of four, and let the breath fall out in a slow exhale for a count of six. Do this for five to 10 minutes, then relax and breathe normally. You'll likely find that your breath has "stretched" and become fuller, longer, and easier.

Being well-rested and calm helps you do everything better—think, work, cope with stress, be a good partner, be a good parent—and it aids everything from immunity to hormones to brain power. A bedtime ritual is an easy, pleasant addition to your nighttime routine that could make a big difference.

Props for stretching and inverting

Inversions, aka being upside down, are anti-aging. They improve lymphatic drainage, up your energy and mental stamina, and lift your mood. Going upside down shifts organs a bit and reverses blood flow, which increases circulation to spots that normally don't get as much "nourishment," including the brain.

Inversions also improve digestion and can relieve pain in the extremities. And they make you feel fantastic—high in the best, most natural way. You don't necessarily need props to help you invert; any position where your head is lower than your heart counts (standing and touching your toes, for example). But props make inversions more fun and make it easier to stay upside down for longer.

A backbender, such as the Backbending Bench from YogaProps.com, not only gets your head lower than your heart but also reverses some of the front-of-body tightness caused by sit-down jobs. It gently supports your body and allows you to open your hip flexors, belly, chest, and shoulders (which take on a lot, especially if you work hunched over a laptop).

If you're a fan of headstands, there are supportive stools like the FeetUp Headstand Yoga Stool, from Yogamatters.com, that let you invert with no pressure on the head; in general, when doing a headstand, you should be taking the weight in your forearms, not in your head and neck. It's strenuous without support (and can result in neck compression, which is not good). Props can prevent that.

These gadgets are something to consider but are by no means required. Hanging off the edge of the bed like you did when you were a kid is an inversion. A standing forward bend is an inversion. So is lying on your back on the floor (or the bed) with your legs up, resting on the wall—or a variation, lying on your back with your lower legs resting on the seat of a chair. This is a great pose to welcome yourself home with, after work and before dinner. It can really lift your mood. You can do it with your partner, catching up on your day while the pressure flows out of your feet. It's a nice way to decompress.

This is all part of a general policy to counterstretch whenever you can—to wash away a static pose with the opposite shape. If you're on your feet all day, go upside down for a few minutes. If you're rounded over a keyboard most of the time, lie down on the floor and arch your back over a yoga block or a rolled-up blanket.

Keeping back and front muscles in shape—both stretched and strong—will protect you from pain and help your posture. We've all seen what age can do to posture; as muscles tighten, shoulders round. But it's not inevitable. Like a lot of things, good posture just takes more effort as you get older: more attention (are the settings on your work chair ergonomically correct?); more breaks (take a walk, cop a squat, shake out your arms); more movement all day long; more stretching, more foam-rolling, more strengthening. And more awareness, so you notice when you're slumping and correct it. It's worth it. Nothing makes you look and feel younger than healthy posture and a nice easy gait.

Try CBD instead

Before you reach for alcohol, Ambien, Xanax, Aleve, Advil, Lexapro, or Bengay, consider high-quality CBD.

We're still in the early stages of widespread CBD use, and there's definitely guesswork involved in application. Doctors are unsure about dosages. We don't yet know how each separate strain affects different people. The field is unregulated, so it's hard to determine whether you're getting high-quality product. Different people have different reactions to different brands. In the wellness community, we still have a lot to learn.

What we *do* know is that CBD is effective in temporarily relieving a number of discomforts that usually bring people to the medicine cabinet; it's particularly good for insomnia, stress, anxiety, and inflammation. And it's better for your body than the meds we so often reach for. So we encourage you to try it. Here's some guidance.

- **Quality.** Be sure to get organic, unsprayed CBD. Some of the brands we like are Charlotte's Web, the Alchemist's Kitchen, and Flora + Bast.

- **Delivery system.** CBD can be administered a few ways. It comes as a liquid oil, with a dropper; in salves and ointments; and in edibles like gummies. Edibles are the slowest delivery system. For stress or anxiety, liquids seem to work best. You take CBD oil under the tongue, and it goes straight into the bloodstream, so you feel its effects quickly; liquid oil is also good for general inflammation and pain. For joint pain or muscle aches, topical salves and ointments are effective. There's also smokable CBD, and while we don't encourage smoking, it's the quickest delivery system; for a panic attack, it can bring relief in seconds.

- **Dosage.** This is not yet an exact science. Dosage depends on body type, tolerance (which you don't know till you try a product), and even brand. Start low (at the low end of the recommendations below), and go slow. Everybody's different. A certain dosage may reduce anxiety, but a little more may agitate you. So you need to experiment. We've seen different people experience vastly different reactions to the same strains and dosages. CBD comes in different concentrations; for a first go-round, opt for a low concentration. If that doesn't do the trick, move up as needed.

Chronic discomfort or inflammation: 5–20 mg CBD per day

Anxiety: 10–40 mg CBD per day

Sleep issues: 40–160 mg CBD per day

The CBD we're talking about is the type with no THC. In states where it is legal, CBD with THC is available over the counter; this is more effective than plain CBD for many symptoms. But at press time, in most places, it needs to be prescribed by a doctor. As for delivery systems, here's what we know right now.

Good	Bad
CBD oil (or CBD/THC oil)	Smoking
Edibles	Vaping

Deep sleep to the rescue

"**Erin, 48,** comes to see me because she's exhausted. She's been putting on weight, despite eating well and exercising; she can't focus and finds that she's getting sick a lot. Every time she gets over a cold, she's hit with another one. If someone at work has a bug, she catches it. She's sniffling when I see her. Her eyes are red and tired.

I ask about her bedtime routine. She says she goes to sleep late during the week. Dinner is always on the late side because of her tween kids' schedules—sports, theater rehearsals. After Erin says goodnight to her kids, she watches TV with her husband, sometimes falling asleep in the living room. If she doesn't pass out on the couch then wake up needing to pee and stumble upstairs, she gets in bed late, around midnight. She's too wiped out to have sex. She's unhappy about that, and it's causing tension in her relationship.

I tell Erin to eat dinner earlier and get to bed right after the kids go to sleep. I tell her to turn off all screens by 10 p.m. at the latest and to have a real transition period—take a bath, listen to calming music, dim the lights. To try to prepare for sleep and not use her iPad in bed. And then first thing in the morning, to get outside in the sunshine. I ask her how she can fit in that last point. She says she can park a little farther from the office and walk the rest of the way. This will also help her get more sunshine—her vitamin D level is low. At lunch, she has time to sit in the sun for 20 minutes, arms and legs exposed. She follows my advice, going to bed and waking up at about the same time every day; she darkens her room completely; she kicks the dog out of the bed, because he wakes her and her husband when he moves around. Eventually Erin is getting seven to eight hours of sleep a night.

Gradually she begins to feel more rested. About a month later, she sees on her Oura Ring (a personal tracking device I recommend to her) that her sleep cycles have improved. I give her vitamin D supplements to help with her immune system, and she continues to get as much daytime sunshine as she can. With these more restorative nights, she finds that her energy is up. She and her husband are doing great. And Erin is no longer catching a cold every time someone in the office sneezes. She's stronger, more energetic, and feeling better about everything."

THINK ABOUT IT:

- How many hours' sleep do you generally get?

- When was the last time you had a great night's sleep?

- How radically does your weekend sleep schedule differ from your weekday schedule?

- How do you prepare for sleep? What's the typical breakdown of your last waking hour of the evening?

- When you get up in the morning, do you feel refreshed?

- Do you experience an energy dip around the same time every day?

- What else do you do to restore and refresh on a daily level? How about on a weekly level?

FOCUS ON FOOD

———

Upping the quality of what you eat,
actively cultivating a healthy gut,
adapting to evolving nutrition needs,
and replacing misinformation with
truth—backed by science

Food in its natural state

When possible, you should be eating almost exclusively food that's fresh, natural, and real—as in, the kind of thing that will go bad if it's not refrigerated. Not food in boxes and cans, not food in sealed bags with an eerily long shelf life. It's such a simple concept, and yet it needs to be stated, because we're programmed to do otherwise.

"Processed" food is not just the junky stuff we associate with unhealthy eating. It's most packaged foods, anything with a nutrition label. It's a lot of what we ordinarily eat, and we encourage you to move away from it toward truly fresh food in its natural, messy, just picked, just fished, just churned state. Eat as close to nature, as close to the source, as you can.

Often the problem is in what we're doing to our food rather than the food itself. You want to find the least altered, least sprayed, cleanest food, in all categories. Organic is important, especially for certain crops. See the Environmental Working Group's Shopper's Guide to Pesticides in Produce (at EWG. org) for the dirtiest and cleanest fruits and vegetables, so you can make smart choices.

Local food from a farmers' market is great because you can talk to farmers and learn about their practices and because local food is more likely to have been harvested closer to the time you buy it—it hasn't endured lengthy trucking.

The more altered your food is—through exposure to pesticides like glyphosate, through manipulating and injecting, through refining, through extended storage—the more potentially problematic it can be to the immune system and your entire body. A lot of food in the United States has been severely messed with.

The fresher and cleaner your food, the better it is at delivering the micro- and macronutrients your body needs. It's not just produce, like greens, vegetables, legumes, and fruit, that matters. You also want the best, cleanest possible options in other categories: raw nuts; eggs from pasture-raised chickens; meat and dairy from animals allowed to roam, fed clean grass, and raised without antibiotics.

Your diet should be super high in non-starchy vegetables and other greens, and full of variety. Different vegetables have different nutrients. If you have a routine and love to eat the same thing every morning, make sure to mix things up later in the day. Following the seasonal lead of your region is a very easy way to get a range of nutrients without having to think too much about it—as is eating a rainbow of colors. Deeply pigmented veggies are packed with nutrients.

Read labels and pay attention to ingredients, but most of the food you buy should not even *have* labels. Some terms that are hollow or worse when it comes to packaged foods include "diet," "lite," "reduced calorie," "low-fat," "low-salt," "natural," and "fat-free." Don't believe the hype. "Multigrain," "no trans fats," "made with natural flavors"—these terms too are pretty meaningless. Don't be duped by cereals that claim

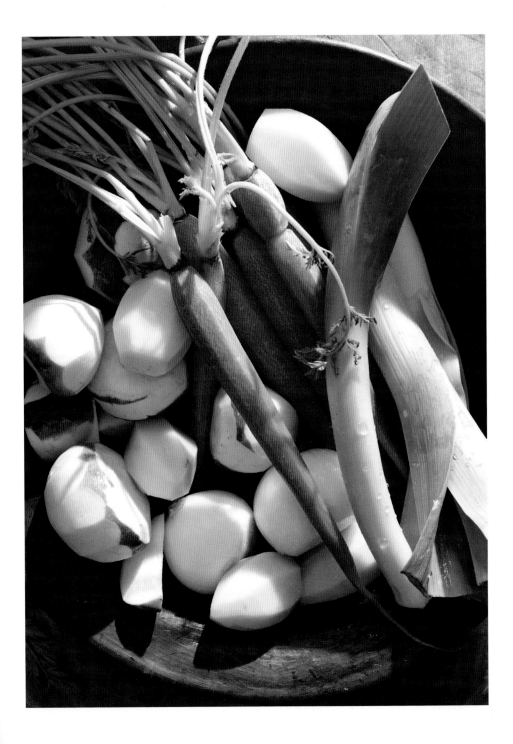

to be "heart-healthy." You know what's really heart-healthy? Not eating cereal. "No added sugar" often means something worse—like the artificial sweetener aspartame. "Gluten-free" is hardly the only thing that matters on a food packed with sweeteners and refined carbs.

Eat mostly fresh stuff—grass-fed and grass-finished meat and wild fish, fresh organic vegetables, raw nuts and simple nut butters, legumes, and some fruits. Go for whole milk, not 2 percent; full-fat yogurt; and good organic dark chocolate that's at least 80 percent cacao rather than processed "low-fat" cookies that are full of chemicals. Compare Skippy peanut butter to an organic brand that contains only one ingredient (peanuts!). Begin to tweak your shopping habits. We're brand-loyal to the core, and it takes a conscious effort to rethink a pantry and fridge.

Practice for a weekend. Fresh vegetables, meat that hasn't been treated, pasture-raised and pasture-finished eggs, an occasional piece of fruit—no refined sugar, no grains. Note how often you're tempted to reach for a box or a bag or a can. Watching your habits for a couple of days is instructive and motivating. Of course, there will be times in life when you can't necessarily shop fresh; but let those be the exception, not the rule.

Training your body to run on fats, not carbs

Most of us are carb-adapted, meaning our bodies use carbs for energy. But carb energy peaks quickly, then sends you crashing. Your body then craves more quick energy—it longs for bread, sugar, pasta. When you eat that stuff, the cycle continues, with your body craving food that's not very nutritious, experiencing a surge of energy, then feeling depleted. This is obviously not a good way to live. And it's especially serious after age 45 or so, because most people become increasingly carbohydrate intolerant, meaning the body doesn't metabolize carbs as efficiently as it once did. This is why the risk of diabetes goes up. Starchy foods also cause inflammation (see page 112) and, no surprise, weight gain, especially in the belly region.

The solution is to change your eating behaviors so your body becomes fat-adapted; that is, it gets in the habit of using fats rather than carbs for energy. This is achieved by eating lots of leafy greens and healthy natural fats, some protein, and very few carbs. So nuts, salad, eggs, avocado, non-starchy veggies, grass-fed meat, fatty fish.

Healthy fats are a much better source of fuel than starch is. Fat burns slowly and evenly. It keeps you energized for a long time and allows your blood sugar to stay steady. When your body is getting its energy from natural fats, you don't experience radical peaks and valleys. So becoming fat-adapted instead of carb-adapted is kind of life-changing.

It's also easy to eat a lot less with this plan, which is (literally) the most important change for aging well (see page 19). Leptin, a hormone that regulates hunger and feelings of satiety, is disrupted by too many sweets and starches. When you cut out those foods, you're likely to feel full sooner.

As your body adjusts to smaller meals high in natural fats, which will take a few weeks, you'll notice changes: Cravings may fade or disappear, you're probably going to be less hungry, and your energy will likely be steady throughout the day.

A little clarification: We're not saying all carbs are bad. Technically speaking, everything apart from protein or fat is a carb. We're talking about cutting *refined* carbs and *starchy* carbs: bread, pasta, snack food, rice and other grains, potatoes, corn. Starch should not be an everyday thing, unless you're amazing at limiting yourself to a tiny serving. But research shows that carbs are actually physically addictive: "Doing carbs" releases some of the same brain chemicals as doing drugs, so it's extremely difficult to have only a little bit of pasta (as if you needed scientific backup for this). Keeping starch off the plate is probably going to be easier and more effective. Out of sight, out of mind.

Here are some motivators. If one of these points speaks to you, use it as a reminder (even a mantra) to stay on track.

- The nutrients you need are in fats, proteins, and vegetables, not in starchy carbs.

- When you're carb-dependent, your blood sugar and energy spike and crash. This feels lousy. When you're fat-adapted, your body functions smoothly.

- Refined and starchy carbs are calories devoid of nutrients, and you want every bite you consume to be nutrient-dense.

Old habits can be difficult to change. A lot of us were raised with three kinds of food on the dinner plate (meat, vegetables, starch), and dinner doesn't feel like dinner without that third food. A solution we've found to be effective: Replace the starch with a healthy fat—a few slices of avocado, a dollop of herbed full-fat yogurt, a bit of fresh mozzarella—and soon you won't even miss it. Or sub in cauliflower rice or cauliflower mash. It has a satisfying starchy quality, without the negative metabolic effects of pasta or rice. Also consider grain-free almond-flour pasta (we like Cappello's). Almond-flour pasta is preferable to pastas made from chickpeas, lentils, or black beans because it's lower in starch.

Two good meals a day

It could be said that when it comes to aging well, breakfast is the *least* important meal of the day. Short fasts, which, as we explained, are so beneficial, are easy to accomplish if you just cancel breakfast. Even on days when you're not officially fasting, it makes sense to think in terms of two meals a day rather than three. Less food means less work for the body, less processing, less energy devoted to digesting and sorting, which leaves more energy for other things, like repairing and rebuilding. Also, fasting is another one of those "mild stresses" on the body that deliver beneficial hormetic effects (enduring a little stress makes you stronger).

Thinking in terms of two meals supports this plan and, frankly, frees up time in your schedule. Breakfast doesn't need to be the meal you skip. It could be dinner. The important thing is to consume the bulk of your food in the middle of the day, not when you wake up, and not very close to bedtime—try to end your last meal about three hours before going to bed whenever possible.

A two-meal pattern tends to become more doable as we age because of lifestyle changes. If you're a parent, the kids may be grown or in their teens, with independent schedules. You're no longer regularly called upon to put three meals a day on the table, which lets you accommodate your own needs with a bit more ease.

This isn't the kind of thing you need to be super strict about. Food as a centerpiece of family life or socializing is important. As we've said, sharing a meal with loved ones offers nourishment for the soul, and this too is an important part of aging well. So two meals a day isn't a hard-and-fast rule. But it's a good default.

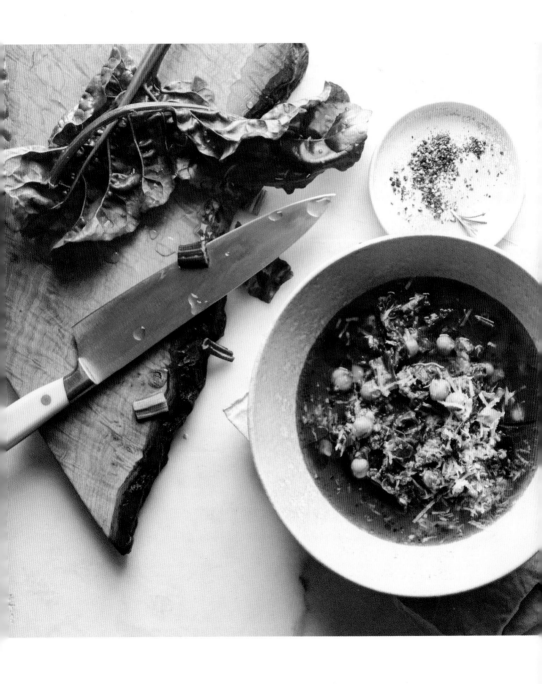

The other key component here is portion size. We live in a country of giant servings. It's out of control. Even when you're eating only two meals a day, you want to keep those meals fairly small and nutrient-dense. The trick of using smaller plates is not new but is really effective: Store away those giant dinner dishes, and dine off of "salad" plates instead. The dimensions naturally keep meals down to a healthy size. Eat till your hunger goes away, not till you're full—and pause before you consider seconds. Take this mind-set with you when you're eating out too. In a restaurant, split dishes with your companion or order from the starters menu and skip the mains. If you find yourself with a big plate of food in front of you, eat half and bring home the rest for the next day.

See what it feels like to eat less. You might discover that you feel lighter and more energetic. And as we explained in the previous chapter, the simple act of reducing your intake of food can have profound effects on your health.

It's not just the food, it's the oil

There are certain problematic oils widely used in cooking that are wreaking havoc on your system. These so-called "vegetable" oils are terrible, and they're everywhere: in the delicious panfried dumplings from the lunch place near your office, in the steak burrito at that somewhat healthy fast-casual chain, in the fries at a good French restaurant.

Canola oil is one of them. Many people mistakenly believe it's healthy because it's low in saturated fat; in reality, it's awful, as are safflower, sunflower, soybean, corn, and anything named "vegetable" oil (which, incidentally, contains no vegetables). All are highly refined and high in omega-6s (that's bad), and many are genetically modified. When heated, they release highly reactive unstable molecules—tiny particles that get into the bloodstream and cause inflammation, which wears you down from the inside, aging your organs before their time. A recent study by the University of California shows that soybean oil, the most common oil used in the United States, causes genetic changes in the brain.

This is easy to work around at home: Don't use any of the vegetable and seed oils listed above. You have plenty of great options to work with. As you probably already know, one of the best is extra-virgin olive oil, which is full of health-boosting polyphenols. Be sure you're getting the good stuff—there have been massive instances of fraud on olive oil shelves. Much like the word "organic," the language that once ensured high-quality extra-virgin olive oil ("first pressing," "from Italy") has become unreliable and somewhat meaningless. Shop reputable brands, focus on freshness, and check dates. Olive oil should come in a dark glass bottle (which protects it from sunlight damage) and should be no more than 18 months old. Think of it as perishable; move through a bottle in three to four weeks.

Some people think that because its smoke point is fairly low, extra-virgin olive oil is not great for cooking. That isn't true. It does have a low smoke point, but the polyphenols compensate for any damage caused to the oil when heated. Uncooked olive oil is especially beneficial to the body. So drizzle it generously on everything—salads, soups, meat.

Other plant-derived oils we recommend for cooking are avocado oil, virgin coconut oil (unbleached and not "deodorized"), and unrefined palm oil (we should mention that some players in the palm oil industry have devastated the rainforest; you can find ethically sourced palm oil with some research).

We're also in favor of cooking with animal fats, believe it or not, as long as the animal has been raised on grass, treated well, and not injected with hormones. Good animal fats are healthy to cook with because they're saturated fats and therefore don't oxidize (and cause inflammation) when heated. Some good fats in this category are grass-fed butter, lard, beef tallow, goose and duck fat (very rich and flavorful), and grass-fed ghee (ghee is butter that's been clarified—heated and separated, with the milk proteins removed).

It's easy to stick with healthy oils in your own food prep. The tricky part is avoiding problematic oils at restaurants or in snack foods. You just don't know what you're eating in restaurants, and you should assume that most dishes have been prepared using a problematic oil. One solution when eating out is to choose foods that don't involve cooking oils at all, from steamed vegetables and roast chicken to sushi to steak and salad (dress with olive oil and vinegar).

Packaged snacks are often made with canola or other inflammatory vegetable oils—just one of many reasons to avoid them. Read labels on crackers, pretzels, and chips; we bet you can't find one that doesn't contain one of the offending oils (to review, that's canola, safflower, sunflower, soybean, corn, and vegetable oil). Skip these snacks in favor of real food: raw nuts, a handful of berries, guacamole, fresh hummus with vegetables—you get the picture.

Eggs are a natural multivitamin

Don't believe negative talk about eggs. Really fresh high-quality eggs are a great source of protein, natural fat, vitamins, and minerals. "Superfood" is an overused term, but eggs actually earn the title. They're loaded with key nutrients like choline—essential for brain health and often deficient in plant-based diets—and lutein and zeaxanthin, which support eye health. For most people, it's fine to consume two good-quality eggs a day.

Spend more to get the best-quality eggs you can find. The language you're looking for is "hormone-free and pasture-raised" ("free range" used to mean something, but now it really doesn't). This is currently your best shot at ensuring that your eggs come from chickens that have been properly nourished.

Boiled or poached is the best possible way to eat eggs, but scrambled or fried in good butter, olive oil, or another healthy natural fat is fine too. When you're eating out, it's safe to assume that the fat used to cook eggs is not the best. So for breakfast at the coffee shop, it's smartest to go with boiled or poached.

Since the quality of eggs is so important, buy your eggs as close to the source as possible. Best is a farmers' market, where you can talk to the farmer. At the supermarket, look for local brands that are hormone-free and pasture-raised. Good eggs are flavorful and satisfying, with yolks that are often a deep yellow-orange. You'll notice the difference.

Less meat and cheese; more nuts and beans

Recent research tells us that as we age, we should be getting more of our protein from plants and less from animals. It's about those longevity genes AMPK and mTOR, which are important nutrient sensors. mTOR controls a number of cell functions, including cell growth and cell proliferation. For younger people who are growing or whose bodies are in reproductive mode, mTOR has many benefits. But when we get older, we don't want to encourage cell proliferation (cancer is cell proliferation). The goal at this point is to inhibit mTOR. Animal protein, especially red meat, contains high amounts

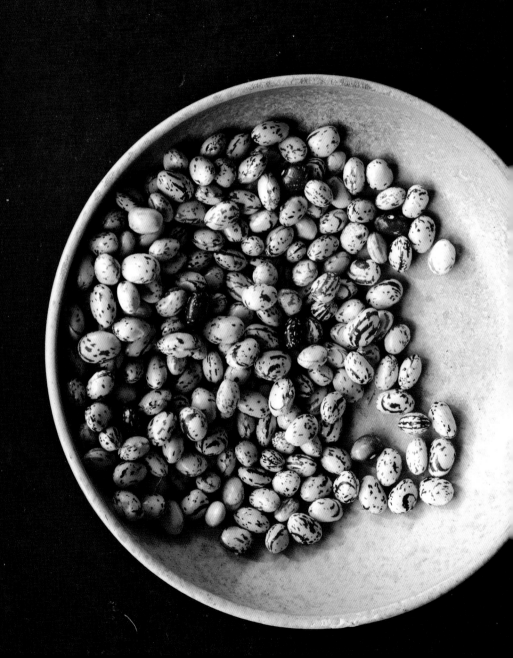

of branched chain amino acids like leucine, which stimulate mTOR. Plant protein does not contain much of these amino acids, so it does not stimulate mTOR as much; mTOR also gets in the way of autophagy (the body's cell-cleaning function). So turn up the plant protein, turn down the meat and dairy.

Here are some of the best plant sources of protein, and the approximate amount a serving delivers.

- **Lentils, chickpeas, and other beans:** 8 grams
- **Almonds, walnuts, sunflower seeds, and other nuts and seeds:** 5 grams
- **Tempeh:** 20 grams
- **Nut butter:** 8 grams
- **Pea protein powder:** 15 grams
- **Hemp protein powder:** 15 grams

How much protein do you need?

Protein can be tricky, because your needs change as you age—and because it's been drummed into our heads that more protein is always better (we all know that a high-protein, low-carb diet is good for weight loss). But between ages 45 and

65, it's more important to eat less meat and dairy than it is to go crazy with protein. A person in this age range weighing 150 pounds needs about 55 grams of protein a day. Most people get this amount without too much effort.

After age 65, protein becomes extremely important. At this point, your body needs more protein, to combat sarcopenia—loss of muscle mass—which is just a natural part of life (see page 124 for more on this). So you want to increase your protein intake by about 25 percent: A 150-pound person who's 65 or over should aim for about 70 grams of protein a day. This, combined with exercise, especially strength training, helps minimize the loss of muscle mass.

Is it better to increase your protein sooner, between age 45 and 65? No. It's actually better not to, if your source, as it is for most folks, is meat and dairy. As we explain on page 88, there are issues with animal protein. Once your body has changed from production mode to preservation mode (at about age 45), too much animal protein can support the growth of things you don't want growing.

The tipping point is around age 65. From 65 on, if you need to eat more animal products than you've been consuming to get the amount of protein you need, so be it. It's very important.

Get eggs and meat from a good source

Natural fats from animals raised well provide excellent fuel for the body. We're in favor of small amounts of meat that come from the right place. The problem is, most animal products have been badly messed with. In concentrated animal-feeding operations (CAFOs), animals are given antibiotics to prevent infection from the crowded, unsanitary conditions (and also to fatten them up); if you're eating CAFO (aka factory-farmed) meat, you're eating antibiotics, which screws up your microbiome. Also, many producers of meat feed cows corn instead of grass, because corn is cheaper. Cows are ruminants; they should be eating grass. When you get a piece of steak from a cow that's been raised on corn, the fat profile is all wrong—a healthy fat has been turned into an unhealthy fat. CAFO fish, dairy, and eggs come with a lot of the same problems. This is why it's so important to find grass-fed and grass-finished meat ("finished" is a critical term, because there are not enough regulations around industry language to give "grass-fed" a reliable time frame—were the animals grass-fed for only a week, and then given corn?). For chicken and eggs, look for the phrase "pasture-raised." Stores like Trader Joe's and Wegmans have good meat. Another great option, as we've said, is to shop at a farmers' market where you can talk to the people who raise the animals. Beef, chicken, pork, lamb—all should come from the best possible source.

If you don't have nearby sources for pasture-raised, grass-fed organic meat and wild-caught fish, you can order online (the company Vital Choice is an excellent online source). For more protein without a lot more food, consider options like bone broth and collagen powder (it's made from the tendons and ligaments of cows or fish and strengthens the same in us). Organ meats (liver, tongue, sweetbreads) are especially nutrient-dense; if you like them and can get them from a great source, then by all means, eat them. These and the items below are some of the best sources of animal protein. Here's what a serving of each delivers.

- **Grass-fed beef:** 30 grams

- **Pasture-raised chicken or turkey:** 30 grams

- **Organ meats:** 20 grams

- **Wild-caught fish:** 25 grams

- **Pasture-raised eggs:** 6 grams

- **Collagen powder (bovine):** 18 grams

- **Collagen powder (marine):** 11 grams

- **Bone broth:** 6 grams

Good salt, bad salt

Salt has a negative reputation, but it contains key minerals your body needs. You want to avoid *refined* salt (table salt), which has been bleached and baked, and the processed, demineralized salt in packaged foods. Really good, unrefined crystal salt, like pink Himalayan salt or Redmond salt, from Utah (sold under the brand name Real Salt), is good for you and essential. Mountain salts are now preferable to sea salts, because recent research has detected microplastics in certain sea salts.

Good salts contain more than 80 trace minerals that aid in all sorts of functions. Sometimes good salt is the solution to a specific health issue. If you're feeling faint or dizzy when you exercise, or if your blood pressure is very low or your brain is foggy, you might need more good salt. If you feel perpetually exhausted, sometimes a glass of water with a half teaspoon of salt is the fix. Muscle spasms can happen because people are short on salt. If you sweat a lot, you might need more salt (and magnesium). Your adrenals also benefit from good salt. And it's nonsense that salt is bad for your heart. As with everything you put in or on your body, it's about the source and the quality. Buy the best mountain salt you can afford (Himalayan salt is easy to find), and use it generously. If you have hypertension and have been told to reduce your salt, cut processed foods and table salt, and switch to Himalayan salt at home.

Sugar is rampant: beware

As you know, sugar is not just sugar. It's honey, agave, white wine, bananas, grapes. It's starchy carbs like pasta and potatoes and bread and even corn. And to your body, there's not much difference, so you want to keep an eye on your overall consumption.

When investigating your habits for below-the-radar sugar, you have to look at alternative milks, if you use them. Oat milk is, of course, too good to be true. Regular Oatly has 19 grams of sugar per serving and 24 grams of carbs. If you can't tolerate dairy but need a splash of something in your coffee, use unsweetened alterna-milks, such as coconut milk or carrageenan-free almond milk (Califia Farms is a good brand). Carrageenan is a thickener that some people are sensitive to.

Bottled drinks—from Starbucks or the deli or elsewhere—tend to contain massive amounts of sugar. They really shouldn't be a part of your life. So-called "energy drinks" are often the worst of the bunch. There are 27 grams of sugar in a bottle of Gatorade and 32 grams in a bottle of Vitaminwater. As we said earlier, there's no reason to ever go near these. A recent study even links them to a rise in blood pressure. Bottled iced tea also tends to be full of sugar. If you buy a bottle of something to drink, it should always, always, always be water.

While some vegetables are sugary, you shouldn't go around worrying about that. Carrots and beets and other sweet veggies deliver fiber with their sugar: Fibrous foods fill you up, so you're not going to overdo them. You'll feel sated way before the sugar content becomes an issue. This is why fruit juice— and most vegetable juice—is a problem. And why it's best to eat fruits and veggies in their naked state when possible. A whole apple delivers lots of fiber, which slows absorption of the accompanying fruit sugar, and fills you up at the same time. The easy rule is to eat, not drink, your fruit.

High-quality tea boosts immunity

When you side-by-side coffee and tea, there's a clear winner. Coffee is fine—it has no detrimental effects for most people, and contains a small amount of polyphenols, so it's mildly beneficial. But good tea is magnificent. Rich in polyphenols, which activate important longevity gene pathways, repair cells, prime the immune system, and reduce inflammation, high-quality black or green tea is powerful. (The difference between black and green is just the timing of the harvest.)

Buy organic tea, because conventionally grown tea is one of the most pesticide-laden crops, and enjoy two, three, four cups a day.

As for coffee, if the caffeine is not affecting your sleep, one or two cups of organic coffee a day is not a bad thing. But if it's interfering with sleep, it should go. The thing is, you might not even be aware of the effect caffeine is having on your sleep. Could be that you're an afternoon coffee-drinker who has no trouble falling asleep but whose sleep cycle—specifically deep sleep—is being impacted. A break from caffeine can give you some good information.

Of course, both tea and coffee can function as a delivery system for sugar, and neither should. If you use sugar or honey (basically the same to the body), taper down by half each week till it's gone from your life. Or replace your sweetener with Stevia or monk fruit.

A small amount of unsweetened nut milk in your coffee or tea is fine, as is cream, if dairy doesn't bother your stomach. If you use dairy, choose cream or half-and-half over milk, and whole milk over low-fat milk—there's less sugar in the fattier options (yes, there's more fat, but we're much more worried about sugar than we are about good fats).

You should also give MCT oil a try. If you're not familiar with it, MCT is a derivative of coconut oil (it can come from other oils too, but most of what you find in stores comes from coconuts). It's a healthy fat that doesn't need to be broken down and processed, as other fats do. MCT is absorbed right into the bloodstream, and goes straight to the brain. For a *real* energy drink, stir MCT into your coffee. It doesn't have much of a taste, but it's a bit oily. You might want to add some unsweetened almond or coconut milk, and whip it up with a small milk frother—this makes for a rich, creamy drink. The combined boost of MCT and caffeine brings a nice feeling of mental clarity. It's a great way to start your day.

What to think about when it comes to faux meat

Many meat replacement products are junky, because they're heavily processed and contain a lot of questionable ingredients: genetically modified soy, canola oil, sunflower oil, yeast extract, unspecified "flavors," modified food starch—the list goes on. Processed foods are never a great choice; eating foods closer to their natural state is always better.

"Plant-based" is one of those terms that's been hijacked for commercial reasons, in this case, by the faux-meat industry. It's meaningless (if you wanted to, you could call Twinkies "plant-based"). If you eat meat replacements, find those with as few ingredients as possible, and no canola oil or GMOs. Impossible Burgers, in the current formulation, contain a lot of ingredients you shouldn't be consuming. The field is growing, and there will be more and more options, so read up, choose carefully, and don't fool yourself about what you're eating. Faux meat may be better than CAFO meat, but even the best options are heavily processed, so it's not going to be as good as the clean grass-fed, grass-finished meat you buy from a great source and cook at home—or a nice bowl of homemade lentils.

Apply the same rules across the board: Eat whole foods, and be really skeptical about anything processed, especially products with a "healthy alternative" veneer.

Conflicts, contradictions, and doing the best you can with food

Changing your personal food culture is not about perfection. What you're going for is a baseline of healthy food habits geared toward aging well. What does that look like? Not too much food; not eating too late or too early, so that your body gets a good long rest from digesting every day; fresh, real foods as close as possible to their natural form; very few grains and refined carbs; more plants than animals. We don't want to say you should go strictly paleo or keto. Better to look more holistically at your habits—shift your food mindset, and adjust how you think about food as a part of your life. That said, we want to acknowledge the inherent challenges in the advice we're giving. Here are some answers that might help.

Are all animal products a problem, or just meat?

Based on current longevity research, all animal protein is problematic as you age—meat (beef, pork, poultry) and dairy are the worst. So you want to limit your consumption of cheese and yogurt, as well as meat. And when you do eat animal protein, make sure it's from a high-quality source. Fish is less problematic than meat and dairy. (Also, if dairy gives you digestive trouble, skip it completely.)

What about eggs? They're animal protein.

Yes, but they're full of so many great nutrients that they fall into their own category. This is one of those tricky contradictions. For protein, the order from good to problematic is plant protein (unprocessed nuts, seeds, and beans), then fish, then eggs, then dairy, then meat.

Is chicken healthier than beef?

It's really about the source. Grass-fed beef is better for you than antibiotic-laden corn-fed chicken. Get the best-quality meat you can afford, no matter the type.

How many times a week is it okay to have meat or dairy?

Try to limit yourself to five to seven servings a week of meat or dairy, and not more than one serving a day. It's challenging, but it's something to shoot for. You'll find yourself eating a lot more vegetables, which is great.

What about fish and the issue of mercury?

No question, this is an issue. The bigger the fish, the bigger the mercury problem. Tuna, swordfish, tilefish, shark, and king mackerel are among the worst options regarding mercury; limit consumption of these "big fish" to once a week. Smaller fish—trout, flounder, fluke, catfish, sardines, anchovies, scallops, local shrimp—are much less of a problem. Wild-caught Alaskan salmon is also a great choice. Canned light tuna is lower in mercury than canned albacore. Shopping online for good fish brands like Safe Catch and Vital Choice can help minimize your exposure to mercury. You can also get your blood level for mercury checked by your doctor. But it's not just mercury you need to be concerned about—now there are microplastics being found in fish. The oceans are polluted, so you really need to be judicious in your fish consumption.

Is fermented soy better than other forms of soy? How much soy is okay?

Yes, tempeh, which is fermented, is a better choice than tofu. And edamame, which is unprocessed, is the best choice of all for soy. It's very important to buy organic when it comes to soy products—most soy on the market is genetically modified (GMO). One or two portions a week is fine, if it doesn't upset your stomach. But you don't want to eat too much soy, no matter what. Why? Soy has high levels of phytic acid, which can affect your body's ability to absorb certain nutrients (magnesium, calcium, iron, zinc, and others). It can also interfere with protein digestion and endocrine function. Too much soy may be a factor in hypothyroidism or other conditions. So don't overdo it.

I thought processed protein wasn't great, but you're recommending it in some cases.

We need to be realistic. The twin goals of cutting down on animal products and getting enough protein might mean that some of your sources are processed. Organic powdered hemp protein and pea protein are good options, as is collagen powder—add them to a shake. Good brands are Vital Proteins, Designs for Health, and Thorne. But eat whole foods whenever possible.

Can I have as much plant protein as I want?

Sure, but eating less overall is a key factor in aging well. So don't go crazy consuming massive amounts of beans and nuts. Processing too much food is hard on the body.

How do I stick with great food habits when I'm at a friend's place for dinner?

Social eating and time around the table with loved ones is important—there's nourishment in being with people you care about, laughing, talking, and eating. If you can contribute to what's on the table, bring a dish full of greens or veggies, and favor that when you fill your plate. If not, just do your best; eat less of the starchy stuff and more of the greens, and don't get too hung up on it.

Of course, food—even at home—is about much more than nutrients. It's about social connection, love, comfort. It can be what we reflexively turn to when we're bored or lonely. One of the difficulties in relating to food as you age is that you simply need less of it. And if you live a life or come from a family where food is really central, you may have to make a concerted effort to change. Shaping your day around other (non-meal) activities—new habits, new rewards—can be a challenge, but it will pay off. We invite you to give it some thought: How might you need to adjust your relationship with food to take the best possible care of yourself as you age? It's a personal question, and you'll figure out the right answers for you.

Seed your microbiome with stalks and stems

Like protein, fiber is a huge part of a healthy diet for aging well. And by fiber we don't mean bran or any kind of grain at all. We're talking about cellulose plant fiber, especially the parts of raw vegetables and fruits that your body can't easily digest. This stuff—also known as prebiotics—is gold for your microbiome. It's the material that serves as food for good gut bacteria.

It's pretty simple to get plenty of prebiotics: Eat the parts of vegetables you normally toss out: the end of carrots, the

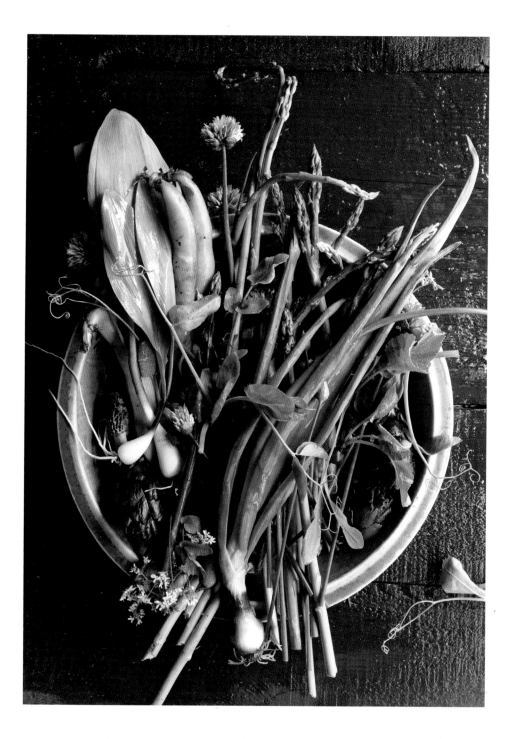

stump of the lettuce head, the stemmed tips of green beans. This is cellulose fiber (aka insoluble fiber). It gets down to the large intestine undigested, where the good bacteria is waiting to feast. Eat things like kale ribs and the hard stalks of broccoli; slice them and dip them in hummus, or toss them into a salad. Have lots of onions, garlic, asparagus, dandelion greens, and chicory root—all great prebiotic material.

The interplay of prebiotics and probiotics is what creates healthy gut bacteria. We're emphasizing prebiotics here because most people don't get enough of them. As for *probiotics*—you probably know you can get them in yogurt, kefir, kimchee, sauerkraut, and other fermented foods. (Food is the best source, but a good supplement such as Activated You Restorative Probiotic can help.)

You have to consciously feed the gut bacteria, the way you consciously feed yourself. We can't emphasize enough how important this is. Your gut bacteria perform hundreds of essential tasks. They break down food, help extract nutrients, produce vitamins and brain chemicals, and have a huge influence on mood. Active care and feeding of these critical bacteria keeps the delicate gut wall nourished and strong, and is one of the best things you can do to improve and maintain your overall health.

A "bad stomach" isn't something to accept

Tending your gut bacteria is one of the most important parts of keeping your immune system strong and your whole body functioning well. And yes, this becomes a little more challenging as you get older. One reason is that as you age, digestive secretions decrease—in particular, gastric acid and pancreatic enzymes. This makes digestion more difficult and messes up the balance of the microbiome. Potentially wreaking further havoc on the microbiome could be certain medications (see page 164), too much sugar and processed foods, and not enough pre- and probiotics. A messed-up microbiome contributes to discomfort but even worse can result in leaky gut—microscopic holes in the gut wall that allow poorly digested food particles and toxic specks (called metabolites) to "leak" through. This can cause inflammation and pain throughout the body (see page 113 for details on inflammation).

The upshot: A "bad stomach" is not something to ignore. It's a call to action. Pay attention. You need to make some changes. If you're experiencing trouble, the following approaches should help.

Try an elimination diet: Cut sugar, processed foods, all grains (including soy and corn), and dairy from your diet for two weeks. See how your stomach feels. Reintroduce possible offenders one at a time, with a big helping of the experimental food at lunch and dinner. This is a surefire way to see if a particular food group is irritating your system. Then (and this sounds obvious, but a lot of people don't do it) *stop eating the problematic food*! Pretend it's poison, and get it out of your life. If you absolutely can't let it go, use digestive enzymes when you eat the danger-food (like Lactaid tablets, if dairy is trouble). But the best thing—and the easiest way to eliminate gas, bloating, and other discomforts—is to simply cut out the food permanently, or at least until your microbiome has improved.

Take bitters or apple cider vinegar before meals. Either one can help with digestion. At the start of a meal, a tablespoon of Bragg's apple cider vinegar (you can mix it into water) or a slug of Swedish bitters (Nature Works makes a good one) stimulates your natural digestive enzymes. Keep a bottle at work too; it doesn't need refrigeration.

Try some antimicrobial herbal supplements, which can decrease bad bacteria and create a healthier gut. Look for a formula that combines some of the following: berberine, grapefruit seed extract, oregano oil, olive leaf extract, wormwood, black walnut, bearberry extract, barberry extract. One we like is GI Microb X, by Designs for Health.

Rest your gut. As a habit, an early dinner and a late breakfast— which we talk more about on page 22—will improve your digestion and the health of your microbiome. Leave a minimum of 12 hours between your last meal in the evening and your first the next day, and ideally 16 hours or more.

Get tested for leaky gut. If you have a functional medicine doctor, you can ask for an assessment called a GI-MAP (gastrointestinal microbial assay plus). This checks bacteria and zonulin levels. Zonulin is a protein molecule used to measure intestinal permeability (aka leaky gut). The test may not yet be available in every state.

Watch your fruit sugar

Although the sugar in fresh fruit is natural and unprocessed, sugar is sugar, so even fruit needs limits.

Favor fruits that are lower in sugar than others; these include raspberries, strawberries, blackberries, blueberries, green apples, grapefruit, cantaloupe, and honeydew. On the high-sugar end of the spectrum are grapes and tropical fruits like bananas, pineapples, and mangoes. In terms of the metabolic effects on the body, a ripe banana is not that different from a packet of sugar in your coffee.

Organic is important as always. The Environmental Working Group (EWG.org) lists crops that tend to be particularly pesticide-laden. The fruits it calls out are strawberries,

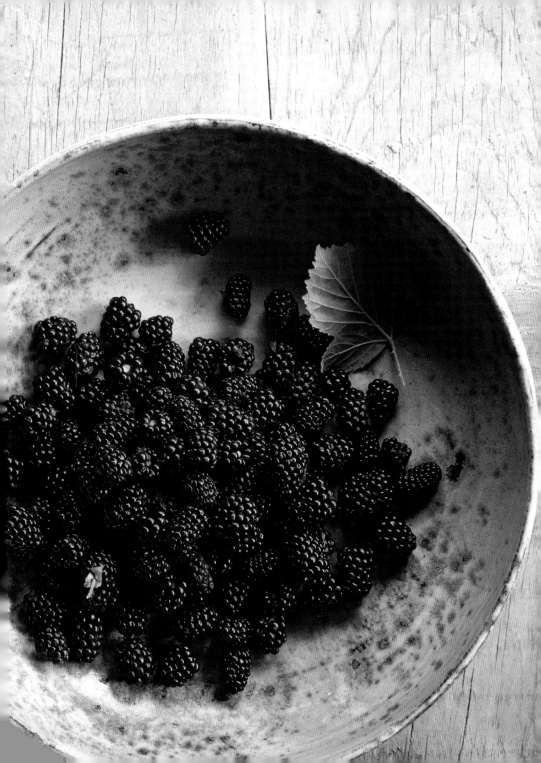

nectarines, apples, grapes, peaches, cherries, pears, and tomatoes. Buy organic or wash very well.

During seasons when there's an abundance of great fresh fruit available, it's easy to overdo the fruit sugar. Fruit is essentially nature's candy, so go easy when the good stuff is abundant: A peach, two plums, and a bowl of watermelon would be too much in one day. Find ways to enjoy fruits in smaller quantities—cut up some fresh cherries and throw them into a salad. Grill a peach and share it as a side to chicken. Toss a few bites of watermelon with arugula and feta.

We've said it before, but it bears repeating: Eat whole fruit, and don't get your fruit in juice form. Juice can be as bad as soda in terms of sugar content. Even vegetable juices often contain lots of sugar, because without sugar, they taste nasty. Have you ever had green juice with no sweetener—no apple or carrot or berries? If you did, you probably would never drink green juice again. Read the label of certain bottled green juices and you'll see crazy numbers—like 30 grams of sugar (seven teaspoons, or almost as much as in a can of Coke). If you do drink green juice, find one with no more than 4 grams of sugar (one teaspoon). When you eat whole fruits and whole vegetables instead of drinking your produce, you get the benefits of fiber, which not only slows the absorption of sugar but also works its prebiotic magic on the gut.

Kombu and other sea vegetables

Eating a variety of fresh foods ensures that you get a valuable range of micronutrients. Seaweeds contain nutrients like iodine that are hard to come by. When you look at the "blue zones" around the world (regions where folks have historically led exceptionally long, healthy lives), many of the populations eat a lot of sea vegetables.

There's also some evidence that in cooking, kombu actually "cleans" other foods—extracting anti-nutrients. Famed New York chef David Bouley says he uses it partly to extract the pesticide glyphosate and other negative elements from ingredients.

With oceans in bad shape, finding a clean source of kombu—or any sea vegetable—is key. Maine Coast Sea Vegetables is a good brand. It tests its wild-harvested sea vegetables for microbes, pesticides, herbicides, petroleum, heavy metals, and more.

You can add kombu to miso soup—excellent for the gut when you use good miso paste (look for an organic refrigerated brand), because of the fermentation process. It's wise to treat sea vegetables the same way you treat fish, which is to say, enjoy them, but have them no more than a couple of times a week, because we just don't know the impact of what's in our oceans.

Inflammatory foods age the body

Many of the good things in life—wine, bread, pasta, ice cream, pizza, fries, cake, corn—cause inflammation in the body. And though you hear a lot about inflammation and its impact on your health, it can be easy to ignore. But it's really important, and it should be taken seriously. So we're going to try to make it a little more concrete.

Let's say you eat a plate of fries. Potatoes are starch, which turns to sugar, so that's going to increase your blood sugar. Because of the cooking oil in which the fries are made, you're taking in excess omega-6 fatty acids, which can trigger the body to produce inflammatory chemicals. (It's not that omega-6s are inherently bad; it's about the ratio of omega-6s to omega-3s. If they're not balanced, it can cause inflammation. Omega-6s are ubiquitous in our food system, particularly in the oils of processed foods. That's why we recommend fish oil supplements—see page 158—they're full of omega-3s.) So now you've got these inflammatory chemicals running through your system. That old shoulder injury that's usually okay but acts up seemingly at random—well, it's now surging with inflammatory particles. Whatever low-level inflammation is always there becomes exacerbated. And you wake up the next day achy and lethargic. In other words, that crummy feeling you have some mornings is *not* in fact random—it's a direct result of what you ate.

In addition, if you're in the habit of regularly consuming junky food, your microbiome is likely to be imbalanced. That imbalance means your gut wall is not as strong as it should be. This could also allow inflammatory particles to leak into your bloodstream, causing irritation throughout your system. You get headaches, feel foggy. You have unexplained fatigue, joint pain, and body aches. You're getting eczema or rashes. You're mucus-y. Your face is puffy. You're gaining weight and experiencing anxiety. And because chronic inflammation is weakening your immune system, your risks go up for cancer, heart disease, diabetes, obesity, arthritis, and Alzheimer's.

Chronic inflammation may not initially produce symptoms, but it's one of the underlying problems of many, if not most, diseases, including brain and mind disorders. In other words, even if you don't know you've got it, inflammation is having a detrimental effect. That's why the lifestyle in this book—which helps decrease inflammation—is so important.

Inflammation is a critical factor in aging. Your body doesn't bounce back the way it used to, and the mantra of "do no harm" could not be more relevant than here: Foods fried in vegetable oils, white bread and pasta, processed carbs, sweetened drinks, CAFO meats—all of these cause harm in the form of inflammation. You're going to feel—and age—a lot better if you avoid them and instead feed your body whole fresh foods, close to their natural state. It's as simple as that.

Bone broth heals holes in the gut

There's no real difference between bone broth and stock—the term "bone broth" was a branding thing. The benefits of the stuff, no matter what you call it, are real, and consumed regularly, bone broth can help protect the gut lining and even help heal damage to the gut wall. You can buy a good prepared brand like Kettle & Fire or Vital Choice, but homemade is going to be even more nutritious and more healing (and also less expensive).

If you already know how to make stock, you're probably set. If not, here's some guidance from New York City chef Marco Canora, founder of the renowned bone broth company Brodo. You don't need to follow a precise recipe. What matters is the quality of your ingredients—organic, hormone-free, grass-fed and grass-finished—and a nice long cook time.

Throw 2 to 4 pounds of **meaty bones** in a big pot. You can use bones from poultry, beef, lamb, or fish—even just the meaty carcass of a whole roast chicken. Cover the bones with **water**, and add 3 or 4 tablespoons of **good apple cider vinegar**. Let this sit for 30 minutes to 1 hour, without turning on the flame. Bring the pot to a boil, then turn it down to a gentle simmer. Cover and cook on low heat for at least 6 hours—go even longer if you like. This extracts the most gelatin and nutrients from the bones. Toward the end, you can throw in some **Himalayan salt**, **garlic**, **carrots**, and **herbs** if you like. Once the broth is done, remove the pot from the heat and let it cool a bit. Pick out and toss the big bones, then strain the broth through a fine-mesh sieve or a regular strainer lined with cheesecloth and let cool completely. When fully cooled, the broth should wiggle like jelly thanks to the high gelatin content (gelatin is the cooked form of collagen)—that's what nourishing broth looks like. If your broth doesn't turn gelatinous, it's still very good for you; just add more gristle to the mix next time (ask your butcher for feet, knucklebones, or necks, or include the skin from a roast chicken; if you're making fish broth, use the head). You can store your broth in glass mason jars in the fridge. If you want to freeze it, leave a couple of inches of space at the top of containers to allow for expansion, or freeze without lids and cap containers later.

When you want some broth, open a container, scoop off and toss the solid layer of fat on top, then warm the broth in a saucepan. (Don't microwave bone broth; it changes the composition of the nutrients.) Crush fresh herbs like thyme or rosemary, if you've got them on hand, drop them into the bottom of a mug, then pour in your broth. The heat will bring out the flavor of the herbs. If you have a small milk frother, you can stick that in the cup and whip the broth to make it creamy.

Make bowls

It's easy to set yourself up to eat well at home. For starters, the old trick of using smaller plates really works to keep down portion size, which is essential for aging well. Also proven: Prepping ingredients in advance so you're always ready to toss together a mason-jar meal for work or a delicious healthful dinner bowl. If you can spend 30 minutes or so on prep as you put away fresh food from the market—wash greens, peel carrots, boil a dozen eggs, blanch some green beans (leave the ends on—easier, and great for the microbiome), steam or sauté broccoli—you'll be set.

With ready-to-grab greens and veggies, you're always poised to make use of leftovers—homemade or restaurant-sourced. Even if you never cook, you can keep the kitchen stocked, as long as you shop carefully (when it comes to prepared foods, choose high-quality organic, lightly sauced plant foods). Start a bowl with greens and protein, and go from there. Here are some tips that will help you get in the habit of tossing together effortless, delicious, nourishing bowls.

Have a jar or two of something lacto-fermented, like kimchi or sauerkraut, in the fridge door (don't let it migrate to the back of a shelf where you'll forget to use it). Fermented foods are great for gut health, and they add tang to your bowl.

For protein, use whatever you've got: hard-boiled or fresh-cooked eggs, leftover fish or meat, canned whole sardines in olive oil, raw-milk cheese, full-fat Greek yogurt, or beans. Regarding dried beans, soaking overnight before cooking cleans away some of the anti-nutrients that can upset your stomach, specifically lectins. But good canned beans are also fine (Eden brand beans are pressure-cooked, which breaks down lectins). Lentils and adzuki beans don't need soaking.

Finish your bowl with some healthy fat. So you don't get bored with your bowls, keep many options in sight: an avocado ripening on the sill; great olive oil on the counter ready for drizzling; jars of raw walnuts, almonds, sunflower seeds, and pine nuts; Greek yogurt or good cheese, if you're a dairy eater.

Add something unexpected. Not required, but it makes a bowl extra satisfying if you have two minutes to crisp up some shallots or onions in a pan. Toss them on top, warm or cooled. Throw in a few fresh berries or bite-size pieces of green apple for a touch of sweetness. Chop any fresh herb you have on hand and add that too.

It all goes back to the gut

"**Julie, 46,** comes in with joint pain, feeling tired. She's already been
to see three other doctors. Two gave her shots—cortisone and anti-
inflammatories. The third was a rheumatologist, who found that she had
a positive rheumatoid factor in her blood and said, 'You have rheumatoid
arthritis. Here's some Humira.' (Humira is a medication commonly
prescribed for rheumatoid arthritis, an autoimmune disease.) Julie feels
sick on the Humira. She starts having headaches and feeling weak, then
develops hives. She says to her rheumatologist, 'Please, tell me who can
help me without drugs.'

The rheumatologist sends her to me. I take a very detailed history,
because there's usually a reason someone develops a problem like
this, and it's often revealed in a patient's story. It turns out that Julie has
been having gut trouble for years. She didn't really think about it—she
was experiencing bloating, gas, bad breath, acid reflux—but what she
noticed and sought treatment for was the joint pain.

I learn that Julie started having UTIs in college, 25 years earlier, and was
given multiple courses of antibiotics. That's when the gas and bloating
began; these symptoms were ongoing and preceded the joint pain by
15 or 20 years.

Though Julie had not really thought about her gut problems—she accepted
it as normal—her digestion was off, and her microbiome was out of
balance for years. The antibiotics had likely caused this imbalance in
her gut bacteria and probably led to leaky gut, which triggered the
inflammation, presenting as joint pain and resulting in her finally being
diagnosed with rheumatoid arthritis.

I give her a combination of berberine, oregano oil, wormwood, and
other antimicrobial herbs to kill the overgrowth of the 'bad guys' in her
gut. I temporarily put her on a low-carb diet—not just gluten-free and

dairy-free, but also grain- and legume-free. I have her cut out nightshades (tomatoes, eggplant, peppers, and white potatoes) because these foods can trigger inflammation in someone who has leaky gut. To help the leaky gut heal, I add glutamine powder and fish oil and tell her to drink bone broth daily.

I have Julie do a five-day fasting-mimicking diet once a month: high in natural fats, low in carbs, low in protein (with no animal protein)—soups and salads only. Julie feels the inflammation decrease radically during the fast. The swelling and pain in her joints subside significantly.

Julie's gut starts feeling better; over the next six months, her inflammation steadily decreases till eventually she has no pain or swelling in her joints at all. Eventually her autoimmune numbers reverse. The antibodies go away, and her numbers become normal. She maintains a low-carb diet, and she's doing great."

THINK ABOUT IT:

- What are the gut problems you ignore? Are you bloated and gassy? Do you have indigestion?

- Have you tried fasting?

- What are the aches and pains you live with every day?

- Have you ever tried eliminating inflammatory foods?

- When do you feel your best, and when do you feel your worst? What did you eat the day before?

LEVEL 4:

FITNESS AND REST

Keep your body in motion, exercise intelligently, and take daily recovery seriously—from sleep to massage to meditation.

Yin and yang your workouts

As you map out your week, plan some form of movement every day and build in variety—balance biking with yoga, swimming with tai chi. The more varied your routine, the better. Variety reduces the risk of injury, keeps your body nimble, and helps you stay motivated. Even within your workouts, you can enjoy a yin-yang mentality. This happens naturally if you're, say, biking over hilly terrain—a hill comes, you crank to get to the top, and then you're back in a comfortable movement zone. Mimic this pattern with other types of exercise—which is to say, don't worry about maintaining an elevated heart rate for a certain amount of time. It's more effective to pop in moments of intensity (see page 49 for more on this).

Most important is to move a lot without hurting your body. Cultivate the wisdom to know what's normal, as far as your body's capacity to tolerate certain types of exercise, and not to resist change—that's the yin part. Also nurture the drive and motivation to do the most you can to be the healthiest you can be. There's the yang part.

Running is okay if your form is good, but I do see a lot of patients who injure themselves running. There are other ways to push yourself that might be better for your joints and muscles, like biking or swimming.

No matter what, let your body guide you in how far to push on a particular day. Be alert: This is helpful in preventing injury and feeling your best. In a perfect world, you'd be able to follow your body's lead on all things, letting it tell you when it wants to eat and when it's ready to fast, when it needs to get in bed early and when it's primed for a tough workout. As much as is practical, listen and heed what you hear.

If you like tracking technology, consider options like the Oura Ring; it can let you know when your body is ready for a stronger or lighter workout by noting your heart rate variability, which is a good measure of healthy function of the nervous system (your nervous system affects everything else). For the rest of us, it's simply about tuning in, paying attention, and remembering that it's much more important to do something physical than it is to do something strenuous.

Maintaining muscle mass is critical

Most of us lose about 1 percent of muscle mass each year after 40. So by the time we hit 70, we're probably working with about half the muscle mass we had when we were in our 20s. It's just a natural part of aging, called sarcopenia, and minimizing it is a priority for aging well.

Until your late 50s, you shouldn't worry much about sarcopenia; as long as you're taking good care of yourself and exercising, you should be okay. Beginning at around 60 or 65,

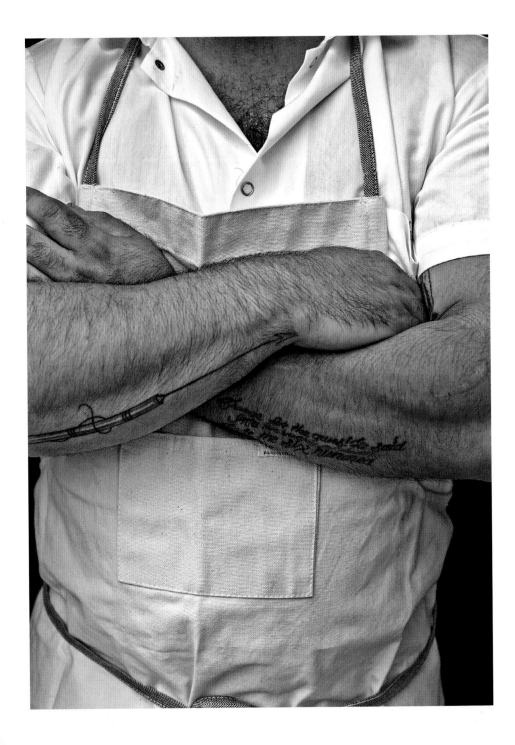

many of us need to increase protein by about 25 percent (even if this necessitates consuming more animal protein).

The other piece of the puzzle is strength training; resistance exercise in your workout and resistance activities in daily life (hauling and lifting) are essential to maintaining muscle mass. Strength training is not just lifting weights. It's any activity with resistance. Resistance can come from stretchy bands, balls, dumbbells, bars, cords, exercise machines, or your own body weight (holding plank or descending into a yoga push-up—that's strength training).

As you get older, you want to be doing more reps with lighter weight. Exercise in a safe but challenging zone where you can feel your muscles working but you don't have pain in your joints—work hard enough so that the next day you may be a little achy (again, in muscles, not joints!). At least twice a week, do some form of strength training.

Upping your strength training doesn't mean sacrificing cardio workouts. Though cardio doesn't necessarily help muscle mass, it increases blood flow, multiplies mitochondria in the cells, brings more oxygen to the muscles, builds endurance, and turns on (or "upregulates") longevity genes. Do both, and mix things up as much as possible. Cross-training is like eating a lot of different vegetables: You get certain nutrients from certain foods, and various forms of movement nourish your body in different ways. Variety also helps you avoid injury, which is often caused by repetitive stress.

Protein and strength training are the key ingredients for maintaining muscle mass, but there are a couple of other factors too. A generally healthy lifestyle is going to help. Staying away from foods that cause inflammation is important. And ensuring that you get enough high-quality sleep really makes a difference. You can also ask for a check of testosterone from your doctor (both women and men produce testosterone). There are two measures: total testosterone and free testosterone; free testosterone is the one that's important. If your level of free testosterone is low and you're experiencing symptoms (general fatigue, a low sex drive), then bioidentical testosterone could be helpful (see page 173 for more on this).

We can't stress enough the importance of maintaining muscle mass. Losing too much muscle leads to frailty, and this is what you're trying to avoid. So whatever it is you like to do—lifting, crunching, hiking, planking, handstands, boxing, swimming, cycling, squatting, pressing, pulling, pushing— keep it up. And take advantage of everyday opportunities for resistance work: moving furniture, hauling the hose, shifting boxes. Functional strength training counts.

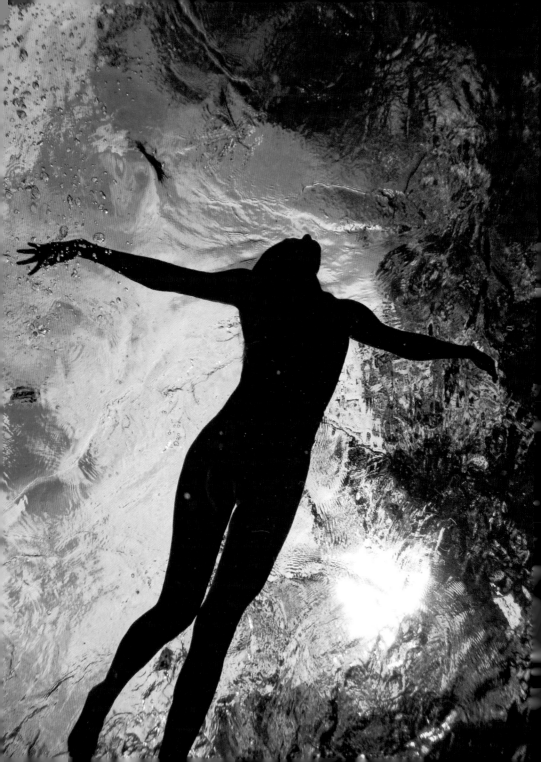

Don't get hurt

Recovery becomes harder and slower with age. That's why it's so important to focus on preventing injury. You can still enjoy a challenging, sweaty workout and get that exercise high, but don't push to your absolute limit. Exercising too hard is a form of stress on the body. And too much stress can not only lead to injury but can also strain the immune system.

Go a bit gentler in general, say to 80 percent of your ability. And if you have a feeling that something in your routine is causing damage, *stop doing it*. Here are some tips to keep you on track.

- **Stretch, roll, and warm up—it's not a waste of time.** There's a reason that a spate of stretching studios have cropped up in the past few years. We're not doing enough stretching, and that can lead to tight muscles and restricted fascia, predisposing you to pain and injury. Stretched-out, limber muscles keep your joints comfortable, your posture healthy, and your gait easy. Stretch before exercise, then start slow, whether you're swimming, biking, lifting, or practicing yoga. Give the body a chance to ramp up. Stretch again at the end of a workout. Foam-rolling (see page 52) deserves another shout-out here. Regular rolling will not only help your body feel more open and less achy but will also minimize the risk of injury.

- **Notice what hurts and why.** It's easy to become used to aches and pains. Your body adjusts to protect itself. You turn your foot sideways on the stairs so the Achilles tendon doesn't have to stretch as much or the knee takes less impact. You favor one arm when lifting something heavy. Investigate what you're accommodating and possibly missing, so you can fix the problem instead of working around it. Because workarounds very often end up hurting something else. It starts in your foot, then gets to your hip and your back and then your shoulder—eventually you end up with a pile of imbalances and discomforts that are harder to untangle and address. A good physical therapist or someone who works with body mechanics (like a specialist in Alexander Technique) can help you figure out what might be affecting your gait, the way you carry your bag, how you do ordinary things like climb the stairs—and note imbalances in your body. The right exercises can help you avoid a cycle where compensating for one injury creates another.

- **Don't wait—treat it now.** Staying strong and agile—and being able to continue to do the type of movement you love—is partly about catching problems before they turn into something more serious. If something hurts and taking a break doesn't fix it, get help. Don't wait. Go as soon as possible. An injury that's not getting better needs intervention—whether it's acupuncture, physical therapy, deep-tissue work, or something else, the sooner you treat it (and the younger you are when you address it), the better. Start with the least invasive form of help, then move to more invasive ones if you have to.

- **Check your form and habits to prevent future injuries.** Any repetitive movement done incorrectly is going to create damage in the body, at any age. But it matters much more as you get older, because recovery is harder. It's not always easy to know what correct alignment looks like while exercising. And even if you do, you can't see yourself if you're not in front of a mirror. Making the situation even tougher is the fact that there are lots of folks leading fitness classes who don't necessarily know body mechanics—and often they don't even offer modifications. So you need to be in charge of your own body. A great gift to yourself is a session with a skilled trainer or physical therapist who can check your form and correct your workout. Ask questions. ("It hurts here when I do this—how can I work this muscle group instead?") Even forms of exercise that have a reputation for being gentle, like yoga, can result in injuries. It's not always easy to find an expert for an assessment, but if you can do it—and repeat the check-in process every year or so—you'll be able to keep bad habits at bay. Minimizing misalignment and the ensuing damage is an investment in your current and future wellness. You want to be able to still do the stuff you love when you're 90.

The hard lesson of overexercising

"**Steve, 65,** has run the New York City marathon twice and intends to do it again this year. He comes to see me hunched over, with lower back pain and shoulder pain. 'I'm walking like an old guy,' he says. 'What happened?' Steve prides himself on his strength and fitness level, and he's shocked by what feels like his body betraying him.

Steve has collected a lot of injuries over the years. He hasn't adapted his workouts to protect those injuries or shifted into a 'preservation' mindset, which is what we all need to do as we age. Instead he pushes and pushes, and then pops tons of Aleve at night.

Steve has particularly tight hips, and because of this, his hip muscles are not firing properly when he's running. This makes the back muscles work harder—it puts an extra load on them. Steve's upper back and shoulders are also tight, probably from years of sitting at a desk. I refer Steve to the chiropractor in my office for some Active Release Technique (ART) massage. The ART helps loosen the hips and upper back. In the office, we teach him foam-rolling techniques that focus specifically on releasing the hips and upper back and tell him to roll daily—twice if he can fit it in. Once Steve gets into rolling and loosens his hips, which he never realized were so tight, things improve. Now that the hip muscles are firing and doing their job, the lower back pain and shoulder pain disappear, as the extra load on those muscle groups lightens. Steve says, 'I haven't felt so loose in 20 years.' I suggest tai chi to help keep his lower back stretched and agile, and he becomes a convert.

Steve begins to modify his exercise routine, namely to stop doing things that hurt. He changes his mindset—stops treating symptoms with Aleve, and instead focuses on preventing injury and taking care of what he's got. We get him off the Aleve completely. He decides that he's done enough marathons, and he gets into biking.

He begins going for weekly infrared saunas and regular massages. He embraces caring for his body in a gentler way. Although he talks about doing a Century Ride (that is, a 100-mile bike race), he's listening to his body more than ever, he's off the Aleve, and he's on the mend."

THINK ABOUT IT:

- Where does it hurt? Do you ignore this pain?

- If you're a hard-core exerciser, do you ever notice that your body feels a lot better the day after you miss a workout?

- Are you honoring injuries and doing something to make them feel better?

- When does your body feel best (i.e., hurt least)?

- What pains have you accepted as part of the normal aging process?

- Have you tried a foam roller? Saunas? More stretching? What's the barrier to any of the above?

- Is regular massage something you can find room for in your budget?

- Does your insurance cover massage if it's prescribed by your doctor? (Check—it might.)

Macro and micro activity

Opt for movement over stasis whenever you can. Shift positions at work—or anywhere you find yourself "stuck" for long periods of time. Some people say a standing desk is the solution, but if you stand in one spot for eight hours, that's not much better than sitting still for eight hours. The point and the goal are to change positions often and to move, move, move. At work, if you can switch between sitting, standing, and even squatting (try it; you might like it), and walk or do a flight of stairs whenever possible, your whole body will feel better.

Micro movements matter too. Manual dexterity is something we don't necessarily think about unless it becomes a problem. Making sure you mix it up in terms of micro movements—not just typing, but cooking, playing an instrument, gardening, kneading clay, knitting, or doing origami, say—helps keep hands nimble. This wouldn't be the primary reason to do any of those activities, but it's a benefit and might help motivate you. Variety prevents stiffening patterns. Since so much of modern life demands sameness, repetition, and stasis, it helps to keep an eye on this.

In general, using different parts of your brain and body is a key component to aging well: Seek variety in all things, from the vegetables on your plate to the generations of the people you hang out with to the workouts you choose to the macro and micro movements of your day.

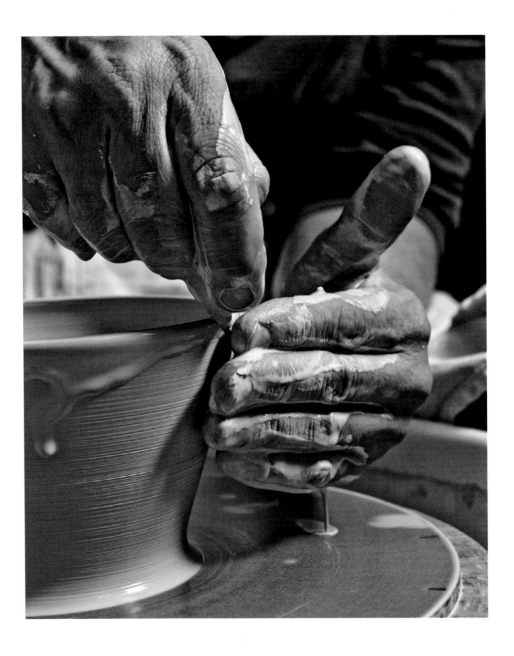

Finding the right yoga for you

If you already practice yoga, you probably have an appreciation for what it can do for your body, and you may have clarity on the vast range of options that fall under the heading "yoga."

For the uninitiated, yoga can range from "restorative"—staying in poses that gently stretch the body, supported by props like blocks and blankets—to Ashtanga, an extremely active practice that involves more push-ups than you might experience in a boot camp class (and yoga-style push-ups are actually even harder than the classic type). In between are popular forms like Vinyasa, often called "flow" yoga, where poses are linked one to another and the sequence stretches and strengthens all parts of the body.

What's common to all types of yoga is the marriage—or "yoking"—of body and breath. Take a moment right now to notice your breath. Is it shallow, landing in the chest, or deep, inflating the belly? Being in a class where someone is reminding you for an hour or so to extend your inhale and complete your exhale has more impact on you—your day, your week, your life—than you can imagine. That's one of the many benefits of yoga—the gift of a full, deep breath.

As you age, yoga becomes even more valuable because it can counteract the potential shortening and tightening of muscles. It addresses the "tech neck" we experience from working on laptops and hunching over phones. It lengthens and loosens muscles that are tight from biking and swimming and running. And it comes with a body awareness and a philosophy that's larger than the practice, showing you imbalances in your body, bringing your mind into your movement (the opposite of running with headphones on), and helping you tune in to the relationship between your body and your breath. For very physical people who love to challenge their limits, mellower forms of yoga can provide delicious balance.

Conscious breathing for relaxation

Breathwork, which you may have heard of, is a practice that helps you manage stress, sleep better, and release tension all over your body. It's simple and easy. The difference between breathwork and meditation is that in breathwork you're manipulating your breath, and in meditation, more often, you're just *watching* your breath—being aware of it without actually trying to change it. Breathwork doesn't have to be anything fancy: It can be as simple as breathing in for a slow count of four and exhaling for a slow count of four. It's exactly what your Apple Watch or Fitbit tells you to do, but you don't need a device to make it happen. Here's a simple exercise we like from breath facilitator Margaret Townsend (TheLivingBreath.com). Try it and sample the effects of a regular breath practice, which can deliver a sense of relaxation and expansiveness, effortlessly transforming a stressful moment or difficult day.

> Sit for a moment and picture your breath as a sort of inner rain shower, cleansing and nourishing your body. Inhale as deeply as feels good, exhale all the way, then let the inhale rise like a gentle wave. Think of an easy flowing cycle. Imagine that your jaw and throat are as wide as your ribs and hips—that you're an open channel for the flow of your breath. Introduce the thought of receiving nourishment as you inhale and cleansing as you exhale, clearing space for the next inhale. Stay with this flow for two or three minutes, or as long as you're enjoying it. Then let your breath return to normal and just sit with the feeling. Maybe let your mouth curve into a light smile (this relaxes the muscles in the face). Notice how you feel.

You can also lie down on the floor or on the bed, turn on some mellow music, and let your breath and heart entrain to the rhythm. Rest your hands on your belly so you can feel it rise and fall (and if it doesn't happen naturally, see if you can send your inhale all the way down so your belly fills up, then feel it deflate as you exhale). Conscious breathing is just a fuller version of the age-old advice to "take a deep breath." It slows you down, feeds your cells, lightens your mood, and becomes a coping tool; eventually you go to it without even thinking. In an elevator, during your commute, on line for the ATM—these are all opportunities to experiment with your breath; stretch it a bit, extending the exhale and inhale; feel where it's going in your body; and see if it can spread elsewhere. Even just 30 seconds of conscious breathing can bring benefits.

A forever practice: tai chi

Adding sustainable healthy habits and practices to your life is the kind of thing that keeps you vital long term. Don't wait. Start now. The fluid, low-impact martial art tai chi, in which relaxation is a core principle, is unparalleled in this department.

Tai chi is a set series of movements, practiced in a seamless flowing sequence known as "the form." It's smooth, slow, intentional, grounding, and deep—and something almost anyone can do, regardless of injury or other limitations. As a physical practice, it has a lot to offer. As with many Eastern practices, its principles also apply as a life philosophy. Soft, yielding, and rooted, it makes a lot of sense, especially when it comes to aging.

There are different traditions, including Yang, Chen, and Wu—some with longer or shorter forms. Don't get hung up on the differences. See what's available locally; if there's a tai chi community near where you live and you're able to learn in person from an experienced teacher, you're probably more likely to stick with a practice.

This is a movement form that makes you stronger with very little risk of injury. Tai chi helps you build strength in your legs and core. It improves balance. It helps you see where you hold tension and learn how to drop it, to root yourself into the ground. It's transportive. And it's something you can take with you anywhere. Once you learn the form (the Yang short form, to give you a sense, is about a seven-minute sequence), you can do it just about anywhere: in the driveway, in a park, even at the airport, if you're not shy.

One of the biggest issues of aging is frailty. It might be hard at this point to imagine becoming frail, but it can creep up on you. Modalities like tai chi, yoga, and foam-rolling all keep you nimble. They're anti-frailty. They can help your body age in the best possible way, and stay with you as a form of gentle, sustainable fitness forever.

Bodywork and other modalities for feeling good

Much of what people think of as signs of aging are just signs that the body needs more (and better) regular recovery. Rather than wait till aches and pains show up, add something to your routine to help the body regularly recover. Our culture treats recovery—sleeping, bodywork, saunas, even lying down with a book—as indulgence. We need to stop thinking this way. If you're active, anything that releases muscles, takes the weight off joints, and circulates the body's chi (aka energy) is crucial to wellness.

There are a lot of things that get the body's chi flowing, but Western doctors don't necessarily look at all the options. Following are some we see great results with, whether for a general boost (a massage once or twice a month is fantastic for your health), to treat chronic pain like arthritis, or for help with a specific injury. Which modality is best for you? That's for you to determine. Personality comes in, expense matters, insurance is an issue, and availability of well-trained practitioners is a factor (a reference from a friend or a trusted medical pro is best). The point is to begin to think about *some* sort of treatment as a regular part of your personal upkeep. Because going that extra mile to support function is part of best-case aging. Here are some ideas.

A massage session with a well-trained massage therapist, regardless of technique, offers you a whole-body reset. If it's in the budget, regular massage can change your life. For specific problems, Active Release Technique (ART) is very effective. It's a massage technique that combines targeted pressure on muscles and fascia with very specific movements while pressure is being applied. For example, the therapist might put manual pressure on a shoulder muscle while moving your arm, so that they can detect and release restrictions throughout the range of motion. ART works well for problems involving muscles, tendons, ligaments, fascia, and nerves, and ART-certified therapists are extremely well-trained. Myofascial release therapy is another type of deep-tissue work that involves slow, sustained manual pressure to release tension. Deep-tissue work can be painful while it's happening, but the results can be significant.

Acupuncture is great for muscle pain, stress relief, insomnia, headaches, hormonal problems, and more. The concept behind it is that the body is a system of meridians—like rivers—through which energy flows; acupuncture unblocks congestion to restore flow (in Western terms, that would be releasing fascia constriction). The needles used are much finer than needles used to deliver medicine—and they're soft and flexible, not rigid. Depending on the point, you may not feel the needles at all, or you might experience a little discomfort that generally disappears in a few seconds. Many people find acupuncture extremely relaxing.

Regular sauna or infrared sauna sessions reduce inflammation and are relaxing for body, mind, and spirit. They can help with chronic pain, like arthritis, and muscle aches from overuse, among other things. See page 55 for more.

Alexander Technique is a system of body awareness. It's all about using minimum effort in carrying out movements and maintaining healthy posture while standing, sitting, and just being. Sessions are conducted one-on-one or in small groups. Alexander can be effective in treating and preventing certain kinds of injury, especially problems from repetitive movement, and is also helpful if you carry a lot of stress in your body. It's a great practice for general well-being.

There's also a lot you can do on your own to address aches and keep serious pain from developing. A thorough daily routine of foam-rolling that gets at all your trouble spots is a lot like massage. Improving your work setup can have a significant impact. Is your chair the right height? Is there an ergonomics expert available at your workplace who can help improve the situation? If you drive a lot, is the seat in your car in the optimal position? For women especially, drivers' seats are not necessarily designed to properly support the body. Do you need a lumbar pillow? A seat cushion? How about your bag? Do you lug around a heavy load on one shoulder? Often it's the everyday stuff that's causing stiffness and pain. Find it, fix it, and feel the difference.

20 minutes a day of something meditative

Here's a question: If something is bothering you, are you able to shut off your brain at a certain point in the day and put it away? Can you stop thinking about whatever the situation is, or does it stay with you and keep you up at night? This is not the only reason to meditate, but it's one motivator. Having some sort of mind-quieting practice helps you find relief from thoughts that dog you—which are likely causing stress, shallow breathing, and tightness in your body.

But there are different ways to quiet the mind. You don't have to meditate, per se, because if that isn't something you look forward to, you won't do it. It's better to carve out 20 minutes a day for a peaceful practice that suits you: something simple that you enjoy, unplugged, without phone interruptions. Knit in a quiet place; play an instrument; listen to music you love, eyes closed; sketch a tree or a person across the way at the park; walk slowly (in nature or even in the city), being mindful of what's around you. Dig in the garden, color in a coloring book, wander in the woods and collect a certain type of leaf; you can change your practice by the day, season, or circumstance, taking advantage of what's around you. Watching fish in an aquarium works. Hunting for sea glass on the beach. Observing birds or bees in a garden.

Take this time seriously, and treat it like an appointment. Sneak off and shut the door, or slip outside. The point is not the formality of classic meditation. The point is to let your mind drop into a quiet place regularly for 20 minutes or so. You'll experience a shift, sometimes subtle and sometimes obvious, if you give yourself this 20-minute block.

And if you want to try to sit and meditate, that's fantastic. We are big fans. Meditation has a lot of proven benefits, short- and long-term. It slows aging of the brain, lowers blood pressure, and lengthens telomeres (those protective "aglets" on the ends of DNA strands). It gives you energy, improves concentration, and helps you sleep better. And it lifts your mood—it actually just makes you feel happier. (If it relaxes you, meditation at bedtime is fine. But many people find it energizing, and for those folks, daytime is best.)

There are great apps for beginners, including Headspace, Oak, Meditation, Calm, Breathe, and Brightmind. You can also find in-person guided meditation sessions at meditation spaces and yoga studios. Meditating in a group with a teacher can be extremely helpful as you develop a practice.

As with yoga, there are many styles of meditation, and classes or apps might mix elements from different sources. Some of the common types are mindfulness meditation, mantra meditation, and loving-kindness meditation. If the first approach or teacher or app doesn't speak to you, find another—don't dismiss meditation altogether. Keep looking till you find the method, voice, vibe that you connect to.

When meditation is the missing piece

"**Jason, 50,** works in finance. He's been putting on a little bit of weight. He finds that he can't exercise as hard as he used to. He says there are all these 30-year-olds joining his company, and he's worried. His identity very much revolves around his success at work, and he feels things slipping. He has aches and pains he never had before, and his golf game has suffered. His sex drive is down. He's feeling like things are not the same in the bedroom. Something's happening, and it's freaking him out.

Five years before, I had suggested meditation to Jason, but he wasn't open to it. At that point, he was very keen on exercise—because it was concrete, and it made him feel stronger—but wouldn't listen to advice about meditation. Things have changed, and people in his industry, especially his superiors, are meditating. Now Jason is opening up to the idea. We discuss it, but I want him to focus on food first, so I don't push.

Dietwise, I say, give me two weeks: I want you to eliminate all sugar, all grains, all starchy carbs, all alcohol, and if you're not feeling better, we can reassess. But after two weeks, he feels stronger. He comes to see me and says, 'I've got my mojo back.' He's inspired. That subjective sensation of feeling better is very powerful. He's ready for the next step. I say, 'Okay, you feel better physically; now we're going to work on you feeling better and performing better mentally—not only being a physical athlete but a mental athlete too.'

I tell him to try the Calm meditation app. To do this every day for 30 days, because it will take that long to really feel the difference. Just 15 or 20 minutes, once a day. When Jason comes back a month later, he's lost 15 pounds, his golf game is better, the aches are gone, things are better sexually. He feels calmer and clearer and sharper at work. I ask how he's sleeping. He hadn't even noticed but confirms that yes, he's sleeping better. Sleep underlies a lot of problems, and sometimes people come in complaining about the *consequences* of poor sleep without realizing that lack of quality rest—including not only sleep but meditation—could be an essential part of the problem."

THINK ABOUT IT:

- How do you feel now as opposed to a year ago?

- What seems to be getting worse? What's getting better?

- What can you add or eliminate to improve the way you feel?

- Where do you think the problems lie?

- What might you be missing?

- When do you feel most on top of things?

- How seriously do you take softer wellness practices like sleep and meditation? What would it take to prioritize them?

LEVEL 5:

DEEPER WELLNESS

Supplements, medical tests, future cures,
and self-tracking for best-case aging

About immune resilience

There's a lot of confusion right now about immunity, especially in light of the COVID-19 pandemic. We've seen this across-the-board fear that people who are older are going to get COVID and die. But the increased risk is not about being older, it's about having a dysfunctional immune system.

The reason everyone talks about protecting older people is that many older people are metabolically unhealthy—they have high blood sugar, diabetes, and/or hypertension and are overweight—which leads to immune dysfunction. It's not about age, though. People of any age who are metabolically unhealthy are at greater risk. It's not a given that if you're older, you're going to have a poor immune response.

But it's true that as you age, your immune system, like all systems, needs more help to stay strong. Younger bodies are inherently stronger. Lifestyle choices have a tremendous effect. There's a lot you can do to keep your immune system strong and to perpetually rejuvenate it. It's everything we teach in this book.

There will be more viruses and pathogens to deal with—destruction of the natural world, climate change, and CAFOs (concentrated animal feeding operations), means we can expect more pandemics. You want your body to be prepared with a healthy immune system.

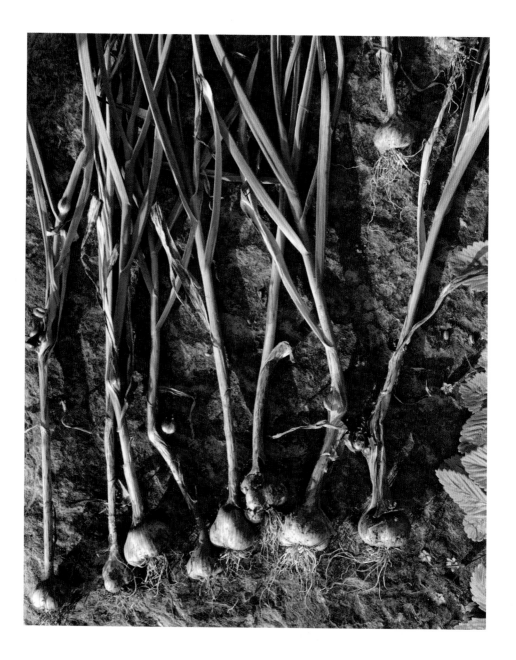

To be clear, a healthy immune system is one that's well-calibrated. One that doesn't overreact or underreact to pathogens. What we've seen with COVID-19 is that the illness can be deadly with some people when it stimulates something called a cytokine storm—an overreaction of the immune response, with an uncontrolled release of inflammatory particles. This can result in severe—sometimes irreversible—damage to the lungs. So while our culture tends to push the idea that more is better, a too-vigorous immune reaction can be just as dangerous as a too-weak reaction. That's just semantics, though. The point is, a healthy immune system—one that's well-calibrated—is not something that exists separately from the other systems in the body. The immune system is intimately connected to the gut, the lungs, the skin. If you're in a good place on blood sugar, blood pressure, and weight, that will help optimize the function of the immune system.

Everything recommended in this book helps you build immune resilience, including calorie reduction, lots of physical activity, fasting, high-quality sleep, stress reduction, socializing—and particularly the points below.

- **A strong gut microbiome.** As we've said, 70 percent of the immune cells in the body live in and around the gut. Actively tending the gut with prebiotics, probiotics, and bone broth cultivates a healthy microbiome teeming with good bacteria, which helps maintain a strong, protective gut wall. This is absolutely key to supporting your immune system and your whole body.

- **A diet high in phytochemicals and low in sugar and processed foods.** Plants generate natural chemicals to protect themselves from predators. These chemicals—phytochemicals—are also immune protective for humans. Different plants offer different phytochemicals, so eat a range. The advice comes back to something we say over and over: A variety of organic vegetables should be the biggest part of your diet. That's the best way to get lots of phytochemicals (not to mention provide the gut with prebiotics and crowd out processed foods). Organic is important; you want your phytochemicals and other nutrients intact and strong, not pesticide laden.

- **Certain targeted supplements.** Vitamin D, curcumin, quercetin, and resveratrol (all explained in detail on the following pages) help build immune resilience and may help reduce the severity or duration of symptoms or complications. These supplements do different things, so they combine well for a synergistic effect. Together they work to inhibit viral replication, regulate the inflammatory response, stabilize the immune response, and regulate cellular defenses.

Supplements for immunity and longevity

Most of the supplements I recommend support the immune system, improve the function of the mitochondria (the energy powerhouses of your cells) and/or affect your longevity gene pathways.

Of course, supplements aren't a replacement for healthy habits. You can (and should) be bolstering function by removing sugar and refined carbs from your diet, getting some sunshine every day, and living a physically active life. Supplements are a boost.

When shopping for supplements, get the best-quality versions you can—without sugar, lactose, or artificial colors. Some brands we recommend are Thorne, The Well, Designs for Health, Allergy Research Group, and Activated You.

Lots of people do well without ever taking supplements. My experience is that supplements don't hurt, and that targeted supplementation is usually helpful, especially for building immune resilience. Although the science may not be quite there yet, I strongly believe that the supplements listed here are beneficial.

Vitamin D (which is actually a hormone, not a vitamin) is critical for bone health and many metabolic processes. It also enhances immune function. I recommend it despite the fact that there's some controversy about its importance these days. Deficiency of vitamin D is associated with certain types of cancer. Have your doctor check your level, and take a supplement if you're low (most of us are).

DOSAGE: If your level is under 30, take 10,000 IU a day; if it's between 30 and 50 (or if you don't know your level), take 5,000 IU a day; if it's over 50, take 2,000 IU a day. Vitamin D is fat soluble, so take it with fat (avocado, fatty meat or fish, nut butter, full-fat yogurt). To boost the effects and minimize the potential risk of toxicity, choose a D supplement that contains some vitamin K (many do), which is good for heart health and bone health. Recheck your level of D after three months; though it's very rare, blood levels of D that are too high can be dangerous.

Curcumin is an extract of turmeric root. It helps combat inflammation, which reduces pain and fatigue, improves mood, boosts cognitive function, and stimulates longevity gene pathways. Curcumin is also found in traditional anti-cancer herbal formulas because it interrupts the normal progression of cancer cells.

DOSAGE: 500 to 1,000 milligrams twice a day. Take it with fat (eggs, avocado—any of the good fats we talk about) so it can be properly absorbed. Add turmeric to your cooking too. It's the number one spice for overall health.

Quercetin is a plant pigment (a colored substance produced by plants) that occurs in small amounts in foods like grapes, berries, cherries, apples, onions, broccoli, kale, tomatoes, and tea.

It's an anti-inflammatory and antioxidant that helps to lower blood pressure, protect the body from age-related diseases, reduce the risk of cancer, decrease viral growth, and support the heart. You can't get very much from food, so it's a good idea to supplement. On its own, quercetin is not easily absorbed by the body. I recommend supplements that pair it with vitamin C or digestive enzymes like bromelain to aid absorption.

DOSAGE: 500 to 1,000 milligrams per day

Alpha-lipoic acid is a potent antioxidant that naturally occurs in every one of your cells, but the body doesn't make enough of it. ALA helps fight inflammation, balance blood sugar, modulate the immune system, protect skin collagen, support the health of your nervous system, and boost the effectiveness of other antioxidants. You can get some ALA in grass-fed red meat—especially organ meats—and vegetables like broccoli and spinach. But most of us need more.

DOSAGE: 300 to 600 milligrams per day (non-meat-eaters should aim for the higher end).

Resveratrol is a polyphenol with powerful antioxidant properties. It's anti-inflammatory, it may prevent cancer, and it's neuroprotective, meaning it's good for the brain. Its effects seem to mimic the beneficial effects of calorie restriction. Resveratrol affects the activity of enzymes in the body called sirtuins (one of the so-called longevity genes). Sirtuins control certain biological pathways and are known to be involved in the aging process. Resveratrol gives them a boost. You may have heard that red wine contains resveratrol. This is true, but you'd need to down 150 glasses a day to get the recommended amount. Foodwise, it's in grape skins, pomegranates, and raw cacao, but you can really get the recommended dosage only from a supplement.

DOSAGE: 200 to 300 milligrams per day.

Fish oil is rich in omega-3 fatty acids, which are crucial to health, particularly metabolic health. They reduce inflammation and lower your risk of heart disease, diabetes, and arthritis. Most people don't get enough omega-3s in their diet (one of the blood tests we recommend on page 167 measures this level). Buy good fish oil that's been tested for mercury.

DOSAGE: 1 to 3 grams per day.

Nicotinamide riboside (NR) supports many aspects of healthy aging. It's an alternative form of vitamin B3 that's converted by your body into a coenzyme called nicotinamide adenine dinucleotide (NAD+), which exists inside every cell. The amount of NAD+ in your cells naturally decreases as you age; this decrease has been linked to illnesses including diabetes, heart disease, and Alzheimer's. NR keeps that NAD+ up, and it also supports healthy brain function and cognition. It works best when combined with resveratrol and quercetin. A similar supplement, nicotinamide mononucleotide (NMN), which leads to an increase in NAD+ levels, has recently entered the market. NR and NMN both do basically the same thing.

DOSAGE FOR NR: 500 to 1,000 milligrams per day.

DOSAGE FOR NMN: 250 to 500 milligrams per day.

CoQ10 is an enzyme that generates energy for every cell, tissue, and organ in the body, boosting the cardiovascular system and cellular health. It's an antioxidant that your body produces continuously but that we tend to produce less and less of as we age. Supplementing helps keep cells resilient and less susceptible to damage (when cells become damaged, organs can become impaired). If you're on statins, then CoQ10 is pretty critical. Statins can rob your body of its natural CoQ10 store by as much as 40 percent. This shows up in a number of ways but especially as muscle pain. The best food sources are organ meats (twice a week will do the trick), mackerel, and herring. You'll also get CoQ10—though not as much—from peanuts, sesame seeds, walnuts, adzuki beans, and vegetables like spinach, broccoli, sweet potatoes, sweet peppers, garlic, parsley, avocados, and cauliflower.

DOSAGE: 200 to 400 milligrams daily for the first four weeks, then 200 milligrams a day to maintain healthy levels. Look for the ubiquinol form of CoQ10.

Cholesterol myths and truths

Myth: Cholesterol is bad.

Truth: Cholesterol is good, and essential to the body. It helps produce cell membranes, hormones, fat. Your brain needs it to function well. It's a vital component of every one of your cell membranes. If your cholesterol is too low, you won't be able to convert the sun's rays into sufficient vitamin D. You can't make estrogen or testosterone without it.

Myth: The most important factor in treating heart disease is to lower high cholesterol.

Truth: What's actually more important in treating heart disease is to lower triglycerides. High triglycerides are usually the result of eating more calories than you burn, particularly from high-carbohydrate foods. Focusing on cholesterol is ignoring the root cause. It's like bringing down a fever with Advil. A fever is your body's defense mechanism, its response to something going on. And when you bring down the fever, that's not really helping your body. That heat might be cooking something away. It's a way our bodies have evolved to fight viruses. Along the same lines, there's some evidence that your body makes more cholesterol as a defense against inflammation. This is only now being studied, so we don't have a definitive answer yet. But the question becomes: Is higher cholesterol the body's compensation for inflammation? And in medicating that away, are you tamping down the body's compensatory mechanism rather than listening to it and treating the inflammation? We need to look at *why* cholesterol might be high and not go crazy trying to lower it without learning what it's telling us. In treating a number that's a result of a complex underlying process, we could be missing the really important information.

Myth: Low cholesterol means you're healthy.
Truth: Our obsession with low cholesterol is confused and misguided. Studies show that people with higher overall cholesterol live longer. In fact, the blood test typically done—the one that measures LDL (low-density lipoprotein) and HDL (high-density lipoprotein) levels—is actually useless. The more important number is your ratio of triglycerides to HDL—that should be as low as possible. Ask your doctor to tell you this ratio.

Myth: LDL cholesterol is bad. HDL cholesterol is good.
Truth: LDL and HDL are not even cholesterol. They're *proteins* that carry cholesterol (and other fatty substances) through the bloodstream. Fat doesn't mix well with water, so it needs carriers to get where it's needed. What matters is not total LDL versus HDL. What matters is the particle size. Small LDL particles can be a problem, whereas large LDL particles are not. The small particles squeeze through the lining of the arteries and can oxidize and cause damage, whereas the larger particles are actually good. The traditional test is pointless. The

better test is an advanced lipid evaluation (see page 167), which measures a number of important risk factors for heart disease, including the quantity and size of LDL and HDL particles. But even if your LDL particles are too small or there are too many of them, the first line of treatment should be diet and exercise. You can also add supplements like fish oil (1 to 3 grams per day), berberine (500 milligrams three times a day), and niacin (1.5 to 3 grams per day—start low, and check with your doctor first). New evidence also shows that fasting (see page 22) can be extremely beneficial too.

Common meds that shouldn't be common

We're not against medications, but we're against the *overuse* of medications. Taking a pill is not harmless. Many people have the notion that "it doesn't do any harm and it could do some good." That's just not accurate. This thinking might apply to many supplements, but it doesn't apply to drugs.

Most medications work by inhibiting certain natural functions of the body (functions that are usually positive), so over time, they're bound to have unintended effects. And generally speaking, drugs treat the symptom, not the underlying cause. If you're driving your car and the oil light goes on, you don't just put a piece of tape over it. You find out why the light went on—what's wrong—and you fix that. Similarly with the body, when you have a symptom, you need to try to ascertain what's *causing* the symptom. Taking a pill usually doesn't help get to the root cause.

The surprising news is that many common meds are not all that effective. So you're shutting down natural systems and piling up side effects and may not even be improving the situation that led you to take the drug in the first place.

There *is* a place for medication. But when possible, we urge you to first treat your body with diet, exercise, quality sleep, and stress reduction instead. Following is some information on commonly overprescribed meds, and how to get off them.

Sleep and Anxiety Medications

COMMON TYPES: Xanax, Klonopin, Ambien, and Ativan

EFFICACY: Benefits are modest at best. Though these meds may help you fall asleep, most increase total sleep time by only 20 to 30 minutes.

SIDE EFFECTS: Risk of dependency, increased risk of dementia, memory loss, mood changes, erratic behavior, confusion, drowsiness, loss of coordination, sleepwalking, sleep-eating, and even sleep-driving.

GETTING OFF THEM: This can be difficult as they cause addiction. Taper off slowly under a doctor's supervision.

INSTEAD: Start with magnesium (see page 54), move on to glycine and L-theanine, then try CBD. For women, the next course of action would be to work with a doctor on checking levels for the hormones pregnenolone and progesterone. If levels are low, supplementing these hormones can often help with sleep. Sleep is very complicated, and what works for one person may not work for another.

Acid Reflux Medications

COMMON TYPES: Proton pump inhibitors (PPIs), such as Nexium, Prevacid, Prilosec, Protonix, and Aciphex, and H2 antagonists, such as Zantac, Pepcid, and Tagamet

EFFICACY: These meds are effective at treating symptoms but don't address the underlying cause of the problem.

SIDE EFFECTS: Prolonged use can cause microbiome imbalances and pneumonia; malabsorption of nutrients like magnesium, calcium, and B12, leading to vitamin deficiencies; increased risk of bone fractures; and kidney and liver problems.

GETTING OFF THEM: Most people develop a dependency and find it hard to stop taking these meds, because when they do, they experience a rebound effect: The body creates *more* acid (hypersecretion), which can cause reflux. So taper off slowly.

INSTEAD: Prevent reflux in the first place by avoiding alcohol, caffeine, and foods that irritate your system. Take the supplements DGL (deglycyrrhizinated licorice) and mastic gum, and drink aloe vera juice. Some people find relief in actually ingesting acid in the form of HCL tablets.

Cholesterol Medications

COMMON TYPES: Statins like Lipitor, Mevacor, Pravachol, Crestor, and Zocor

EFFICACY: They do lower cholesterol, but there are questions as to whether low cholesterol is truly a relevant goal. Look at the website TheNNT.com (NNT stands for "number needed to treat"). This site, started by a group of physicians, reveals the efficacy of a bunch of meds, including statins. Its work is based on high-quality, evidence-based studies, and the site accepts no outside funding. You can search different medications and you'll see how few people are really helped by standard meds. Statins offer no statistically significant increase in life span, and only one in 217 people taking them avoids a nonfatal heart attack—whereas *everyone* taking them runs the risk of serious side effects.

SIDE EFFECTS: Muscle pain, headaches, increased risk of developing diabetes, potential memory loss.

GETTING OFF THEM: Speak to your doctor before stopping.

INSTEAD: Reduce sugar and junk food; increase exercise.

Anti-Inflammatories

COMMON TYPES: Advil, Motrin, Aleve, Celebrex, Naprosyn

EFFICACY: These drugs are effective for pain relief and acute inflammation but are meant for short-term use only. Many people use them for long stretches, with alarming frequency.

SIDE EFFECTS: Long-term use can increase the risk of heart attack or stroke; may cause all sorts of gastrointestinal problems, including ulcers, leaky gut, and a microbiome imbalance; and may also cause kidney trouble, liver inflammation, anemia, rashes, and allergic reactions.

GETTING OFF THEM: Can safely stop them anytime.

INSTEAD: CBD, curcumin, fish oil, bodywork, acupuncture, physical therapy, exercise.

Antidepressants

When it comes to severe depression, antidepressants can be effective and are likely necessary. But for mild depression, studies show that these drugs are not better than a placebo. For moderate depression, they're somewhat effective, but research proves that exercise is even more effective. If you're in the latter two groups (mild or moderate) and you want to take yourself off depression meds, please do so under the supervision of a doctor and taper slowly. Many people experience a dramatic rebound effect coming off SSRI antidepressants (Prozac, Lexapro, Paxil, and others); in other words, they stop taking the meds and feel really terrible, then think they must have been more depressed than they realized, so they go back on. But that effect is just temporary. The body needs time to level off. This is why it's important to have the help of a doctor.

Antibiotics

Obviously, antibiotics can be life-saving, but they're also massively overused. Antibiotics work only against bacteria. Most sore throats and sinus infections are viral in origin. Please don't rush to take antibiotics unless they're necessary—they kill many types of good bacteria too, including critical bacteria in your gut. This can wreak havoc on your microbiome, sometimes with long-term consequences.

Blood tests for longevity

Western medicine tends to look at testing differently than integrative medicine does; there are blood tests for longevity I recommend that regular doctors don't necessarily do. One day these tests will be standard, but at the moment, you have to ask your doctor to prescribe some of them. Another difference in integrative medicine is that the blood levels we consider ideal are often beyond what's standard in mainstream medicine. It comes down to a simple question: Do you want "normal" numbers or do you want numbers for optimal function? We want you to be better than normal. We want optimal function for you.

Many of the tests we recommend on the following pages look at aging biomarkers, which are not necessarily markers for disease, but markers for the *possibility* of disease. They're smoke detectors for trouble. Sort of like a mammogram, they pick up predispositions and warning signs. When you catch a problem early, it's easier to address through diet, exercise, supplements, and other habits. These blood tests are recommended in addition to (not instead of) the typical bloodwork recommended by your physician. And whether or not you choose to test, the lifestyle and diet recommendations in this book should positively affect all the biomarkers below.

Hormone levels. Most hormones will decrease as you age. These are target levels.

- Thyroid-stimulating hormone (TSH): 0.5–2.5 microIU/mL
- Free T3: 3.0–4.5 pg/mL
- Free T4: 1.3–1.8 ng/dL
- Reverse T3: less than 20 ng/dL
- DHEA sulfate: 300–450 mcg/dL
- Pregnenolone: 50–150 ng/dL
- Total testosterone: 500–1,000 ng/dL
- Free testosterone: 6.5–15 ng/dL
- Progesterone: results vary with age, where you are in your cycle, and whether you've gone through menopause
- Estradiol: results vary with age, where you are in your cycle, and whether you've gone through menopause

Vitamin levels. Ask the doctor to check vitamin D, vitamin B12, RBC (red blood cell) magnesium, folate, and RBC zinc. These are the levels you want to see, or eventually get to with supplements.

- Vitamin D: 50–80 ng/mL
- Vitamin B12: greater than 500 pg/mL
- Folate: 10–25 ng/mL
- RBC magnesium: 5–6.5 dL
- RBC zinc: 12–14 mg/L
- Serum selenium: 110–150 ng/mL

Advanced lipid evaluation. The most extensive lipid evaluation and barometer of cardiac function is the Boston Heart

Test. It measures inflammatory markers and cholesterol particle size. It also determines if your body is making too much cholesterol or you're absorbing too much cholesterol—crucial data. It provides much more information than the standard cholesterol test, measuring important heart risk factors like Apolipoprotein A-1, Apolipoprotein B, and Lipoprotein (a).

Inflammatory markers. These pick up nonspecific inflammation in the body and can be an early sign that something is not right. You want all inflammatory markers to be low.

- C-reactive protein: less than 1 mg/dL
- Interleukin-6: less than 3 pg/mL
- TNF-alpha: less than 6 pg/mL

Ratio of omega-3s to omega-6s. You want your omega-3-to-omega-6 ratio to be at least 3 to 1. This is important, and if your levels are not where they should be, it's an easy fix: Just take fish oil, cook with olive oil rather than vegetable oils, don't eat junk food, and don't eat fried foods in restaurants (where the cooking oil is likely an unhealthy oil).

Homocysteine. This measures methylation, an important biochemical process happening thousands of times a day. If you're not methylating properly, among other things, you're not breaking down toxins well. You want a level less than 8.

Insulin-like growth factor 1. You're looking for a number that's less than 200. As we get older, our IGF-1 should not be high—you don't want to "grow" more. If something is growing at that point, it could be cancer.

Fasting insulin. The sweet spot is around 5 microIU/mL. If your number is high, you've really got to watch your sugar. It might be an early sign of carbohydrate intolerance and diabetes. Most doctors say under 18 is good, but you want it much lower, closer to 5.

APO-E4 gene variant. The "Alzheimer's gene." If this shows up in your testing, it doesn't mean you're going to get the disease, but you're more prone to it. Lifestyle habits have a big impact; follow the advice in this book.

MTHFR gene variant. If you have certain forms of this gene mutation, it indicates that your MTHFR gene may not be functioning optimally. Among other things, this may result in a buildup of homocysteine in your blood, leading to all sorts of health problems. Research around MTHFR and its effects is still evolving, but I have seen significant improvements in myriad health problems when addressing this mutation with the supplements: methylated B12 and methylated folic acid.

Testing for these two gene variants is available through 23andMe; this is a much less expensive route to the info than going through a doctor, so we recommend it.

Tracking wellness with wearable tech

Devices like the Fitbit or the Oura Ring make it easy to collect data about yourself. They're useful for counting steps (aim for 7,500 a day, the equivalent of three or four miles), tracking heart rate, indicating body temperature, and measuring heart rate variability (the higher your HRV, the more resilient your nervous system). It's still unclear whether these tools are accurate at measuring deep sleep and REM sleep, but they can tell you how quickly you fall asleep and how long you stay asleep. And they can offer some insight into sleep patterns. As technology advances, there'll be better tracking of deep sleep and REM sleep, which will be valuable. If you're drawn to tracking technology, we're in favor. It can provide useful guidelines, and a lot of people find it motivating: You see where you are, challenge yourself to improve, then retest. There's no telling what's next, but some folks are already going further with tracking tech, wearing continuous blood-glucose monitors that allow them to see changes in blood sugar in real time. This may sound extreme, but once these devices are more affordable, they may become common.

That said, for some people, collecting data is more stressful than it is useful. If you have a history of obsessive thinking, anxiety, or disordered eating, tracking tech is probably not for you. Even if you don't, if the concept of tracking yourself makes you tense, don't do it. It's not for everyone.

Genome testing

You can't change your genes, but you can change how they're expressed, through diet, exercise, sleep, and other lifestyle choices. One way to think of it is that genome testing + lifestyle choices = aging well. We're using data to try to upregulate longevity genes.

As with checking biomarkers, testing your genome offers more information, which can lead to more targeted recommendations for taking care of yourself. There are a number of options; one we recommend is the health test from 23andMe. You'll need to run your report through a separate service for analysis—we like Dr. Rhonda Patrick's site FoundMyFitness, which charges only a small fee. The kinds of things you learn include how to optimize the function of certain genes to boost daily energy levels and whether you have a greater need for certain vitamins.

If you want more in-depth information on the best foods for your metabolism and the best supplements for your body, we recommend a test from 3x4 Genetics or Nutrition Genome, which is more expensive.

The data you gather through genome testing is just one part of your health picture. How you age is going to be affected by the environment with which you surround those genes—stressors mitigated by all the good things you do for your body.

Bioidentical hormones

Sex issues are common with aging, but they're fixable. As hormones change, you might need some intervention, and that's fine. Simultaneously, though, look at lifestyle choices. It's the same principle as applies to general health—you can't get away with the same stuff you did when you were younger and expect everything to function well.

Hormones are like a symphony: When they're all working together, things run smoothly. But when one is out of tune, another may have to work harder to cover for it. For example, food affects the hormone insulin. Too many carbs will stimulate an insulin response. Lack of rest affects your cortisol (the stress hormone). And both insulin and cortisol will impact your sex hormones.

Guys run for the erectile-dysfunction meds, but the first line of defense if you're experiencing changes in sexual function is paying attention to your diet, exercise, sleep patterns, and stress load. ED is usually a systemic circulation issue. It's not isolated. If it's happening down there, it's also happening in the heart and brain. I'm not against ED drugs, but I would rather a guy look for and treat the underlying cause.

For women after menopause, one of the biggest issues is dryness. For this, I never recommend regular hormones, but I do recommend bioidenticals, and my patients love them. Bioidenticals are hormones derived from plants and chemically identical to those in the human body. Estrogen, progesterone, and testosterone are the bioidenticals I'm talking about here (but there are others). They come in gels, creams, pills, or patches made up by compounding pharmacists. The doctor will measure your hormone levels and prescribe a compound that's just right for you. You'll have the prescription filled at a compounding pharmacy. The hitch is that most doctors and the FDA are not there yet on bioidenticals, so you may need to find a holistic gynecologist or functional medicine doctor to prescribe them. In my practice, I've seen excellent results with bioidenticals, and very few side effects. I believe it's a much safer and more effective way of replacing hormones than traditional hormone replacement therapy when levels are low.

Obviously, there's also a significant psychological component to sex. When you're well-rested, when your body is active and healthy, when your gut is in good condition and you're managing life well, when you feel fit and healthy, when you're with someone you want to be with, you tend to feel more sexual. All the advice in this book on diet, stress, exercise, and cultivating a happy life will help support sexual health as you age. And if you're experiencing problems, you might find that something as simple as dropping alcohol will make a big difference.

Intimacy matters. No matter what's happening, don't write it off. If you need some intervention, get it. Don't let a problem worsen, because the quicker you deal with it, the less stress it will cause you and your relationship and, therefore, your health. And in fact, some of these problems require less intervention when dealt with earlier.

Many studies confirm that you can enjoy sex for as long as you want, no matter what your age. As with almost everything regarding aging, it's about taking the best possible care of your body, mind, and spirit—and bumping that up with a little help when needed.

Things that ward off Alzheimer's

Brain-derived neurotrophic factor (BDNF) is a relatively new discovery that we now know improves brain function and lowers your risk of mental disease. It's a naturally occurring protein in the brain that's stimulated by many of the lifestyle changes recommended in this book (see the following page). We have billions of brain cells, and BDNF keeps them thriving and healthy. It helps grow new brain cells and pathways and strengthens the brain cells and nerve cells you already have, protecting them from damage caused by stress. It also protects you from depression and from Alzheimer's (and other types of dementia). BDNF can even improve sleep.

What increases BDNF? Exercise, meditation, quality rest, intermittent fasting, sunshine, green tea, and certain supplements. One is coffee fruit extract, which is made from the berry of the coffee plant; it delivers not only polyphenols (antioxidant-rich micronutrients) but also a brain-supporting chemical called procyanidin. Other supplements mentioned earlier, such as curcumin, omega-3 fatty acids (which you can get by taking fish oil), resveratrol, and magnesium, also boost BDNF. What robs your body of BDNF? You guessed it: stress, exhaustion, loneliness, sugar, and processed foods.

The following all lower the risk of developing Alzheimer's:

High-quality sleep	Cross-generational interaction
Stress reduction	Lifelong learning
A low-carb diet	Coffee fruit extract
Cutting out sugar	Curcumin
Socializing	Magnesium
Meditating	Mushrooms
Regular exercise	Resveratrol
Passion/curiosity	Fish oil
Having things to look forward to	Pretty much everything we talk about in this book

Promising anti-aging treatments

We're not endorsing the treatments below. Although some are promising, they're not without risk. But it's good to know what's on the anti-aging horizon. Consider these items potential add-ons to the larger principles of aging well: eating less, moving more, getting better sleep, developing a meditation practice, socializing a lot, and seeking out joy.

Metformin, which lowers blood sugar, is the most-prescribed medication in the world for people with type 2 diabetes. Many animal studies suggest that the drug also reduces inflammation and produces other cellular effects that alter aging. It mimics some of the positive effects of eating less, in terms of the way it affects your longevity gene pathways. The FDA has approved a study that will evaluate metformin's ability to slow aging in humans.

PRECAUTIONS: Although it seems like the most promising possible anti-aging drug so far, a recent study showed that it may blunt the health benefits of exercise. Other studies have shown it to inhibit mitochondrial function. It also interferes with the absorption of vitamin B12, increasing the risk of B12 deficiency, and can reduce levels of testosterone in men.

Berberine is an herbal supplement that is, in a way, a natural form of metformin (safer but also less effective). It lowers blood sugar and may have anti-aging benefits. The benefits are milder, but there are also no significant side effects. It won't hurt, and it might help.

Hormone therapy is not new, but it's a category that's evolving. Since hormones naturally drop as you get older, the thinking here is that raising levels can have anti-aging benefits. Commonly used hormones for anti-aging are estrogen, progesterone, and testosterone. There are other hormones being used for anti-aging as well. The most famous is human growth hormone (hGH), which is administered by injection. Others include pregnenolone, DHEA, and melatonin.

Rapamycin is a drug that tricks the body into thinking it's in a state of calorie restriction, triggering the longevity gene pathways and autophagy. So theoretically, it can give you the benefits of fasting without fasting. In animal studies, it has been found to increase life span and reduce chronic inflammation. It also has been shown to stave off age-related diseases: cancer, cardiovascular diseases, cognitive diseases. Like metformin, it positively affects the longevity gene pathways.

PRECAUTIONS: Long-term regular use increases insulin resistance, glucose intolerance, and hyperlipidemia (high fats in your blood). In high doses, rapamycin suppresses the immune system, increasing the risk of infection, pneumonia, and cancer.

Stem cell therapy is a good example of regenerative medicine—treatments that help our natural healing processes work more effectively. Stem cell therapy can theoretically enable regeneration of damaged tissue. The research is in its infancy, but a few studies have shown that introducing fresh stem cells, or replenishing the molecules they produce, can slow down aspects of the aging process.

Peptide therapy is not yet FDA approved; research is ongoing. Peptides are basically short chains of amino acids that naturally occur in the body or can be created in a lab. They play a significant role in a number of aging mechanisms (you've probably heard about skin-care products that contain peptides). The most interesting currently is a synthetic peptide called Epitalon. It's a powerful antioxidant that appears to induce the elongation of telomeres.

Cryotherapy is one of many treatments that fall under the heading "cold thermogenesis," which is any treatment that involves the use of extremely cold temperatures for short periods of time. It's usually done in a special chamber or booth for three to five minutes. This exposure to near-freezing temperatures induces a hormetic response (remember hormesis? Small beneficial stressors), stimulates your longevity gene pathways, increases the production of mitochondria, and helps with inflammation. Pro athletes use this routinely now, and cryotherapy spas are opening up all over. Ice baths and cold showers can be just as effective. Some experts say that ice-cold baths are better for the body than cryotherapy.

Sick with stress, cured by a job change

"**Carla, 47,** works in corporate law. She's spent two decades in a job with very demanding hours and intense stress. She comes to my office and tells me she's getting sick all the time, she's always tired, she's depressed and overwhelmed. Even though she's exhausted, she can't sleep. She doesn't have time to see her friends or get to the gym. She talks about how much she'd like to quit her job and work for an NGO, helping people.

I do everything I can for her symptoms: I help her clean up her diet; I give her adaptogens, herbal supplements that support the adrenals (since the adrenal system regulates the body's response to stress). I encourage her to introduce practices to help with stress, to make time for meditation and yoga. I take her off caffeine and other stimulants. Nothing helps. She's still exhausted all the time. Finally, in frustration, I say, 'Why don't you leave your job and go work for a nonprofit in Africa?' She doesn't come to see me again.

Months later I get an email from her. It says, 'Thank you for your advice. I'm working for a nonprofit in Uganda. I love what I do. Two months into my new life, my symptoms were gone. I feel so good.' She talks in the email about how appreciated she feels in her new role. She still works around the clock—that has not changed—but she's valued and respected. She's surrounded by positivity. It's clear from her email that she's in love with her new situation. Leaving a toxic workplace for a nourishing situation had an almost instant impact on Carla's health, and the effects have endured."

THINK ABOUT IT:

- Do you have enough positivity in your life?

- Do you feel loved and appreciated?

- What activities can you add for more positivity and appreciation?

- How does your work environment influence your health? In what ways does it nourish you? In what ways does it cause harm?

- Do you have the power or flexibility to reduce the impact of the harmful effects? What could make things better?

- Is there something you can see down the road that would make you happy? A hobby, a population you'd like to help? What's stopping you from bringing this into your life now? Can you remove those obstacles?

- What's one small thing you can do right now to have an impact that's meaningful to you?

EVERYDAY HABITS

Weaving great practices into your world,
troubleshooting hidden stressors, and
making the aging-well lifestyle real

Do your own chores

You've probably heard about the "sit-stand" test that's supposed to be a predictor of longevity. The challenge: Lower yourself to the floor without using your hands or arms, sit down, then stand up—again, without the help of hands or arms. We can't say if it's a predictor of anything, but it can yield information. Attempting this maneuver offers a nice compact lesson in the relevance of functional movement, which becomes more and more important as you age.

Functional movement simply refers to the movement you use in real life to do normal tasks. The bending and reaching of vacuuming under the bed. The flexion of arms and upper back when you haul laundry up the stairs. Gym workouts branded as functional exercise mimic and exaggerate these varied everyday movements. But, as we've said, you don't want to confine your activity to the time you're able to spend in the gym. It's much more important to be moving all day long—that is, to have an active, physical daily life. So look for and relish opportunities throughout your day to move, in ordinary ways: squatting to dig through a low drawer, stretching to reach a high shelf, hoisting mulch from the back of the car, helping a neighbor move a picnic table. The everyday work of real life—taking out the trash, moving things around in the garage, mowing the lawn—is the kind of activity that keeps the body nimble and strong. And this, more than any other fitness regimen, keeps you young. Don't outsource your chores; when you do, you're cheating yourself out of the best kind of ongoing workout.

Think about your total load of stressors

Your "total load" is everything that's weighing on your well-being—body, mind, and spirit. It's an important concept because it impacts your health in general and your immune system in particular. And taking a holistic view makes it easier to lighten the load with real-world solutions. Look broadly, and jot down thoughts, from money worries to what you're eating. Stressors could include a tough work environment, lack of sleep, not enough physical activity, too much sugar and refined carbs, clutter in your home, chemicals in your food and water, too much alcohol. It's the large stuff and the small stuff: unemployment, difficulty in your primary relationship, a grudge you can't shake, uncomfortable shoes, anxiety from your digital life, loneliness. There's worry about a family member, chronic injuries, working constantly and having no time for play—even a shaky step on the staircase to your basement. All stressors.

Identify hidden stressors too, like toxins in household cleansers and laundry products (see the Environmental Working Group's list of cleaning ingredients to avoid, at EWG.org).

Bleach is a common stressor. Although there are times in the current environment when we need harsh chemicals to keep us safe, we don't need them all the time—and it's healthier for the immune system not to use them regularly. Save bleach for extenuating circumstances, and pay attention to other stressors in the air; use a dehumidifier if there's a concern about moisture and mold, and keep windows open whenever that's viable. Consider toxins in chemical-laden beauty products too—these count as stressors.

The point of "total load" thinking is that many of the things taking a toll on you can be remedied. Go for the low-hanging fruit. Is a worn-out mattress affecting your sleep? Are you suffering from a nature deficit? Are you snacking on processed foods? Is social media keeping you up late into the night? Are you drinking unfiltered water? Are you not laughing enough? What changes can you make?

Elements that may seem unrelated are all feeding into the same machine—you. Each change improves the workings a little bit, and that makes the next change easier. You don't need to get everything right all at once, but over time, see that your total load of stressors gets smaller and smaller.

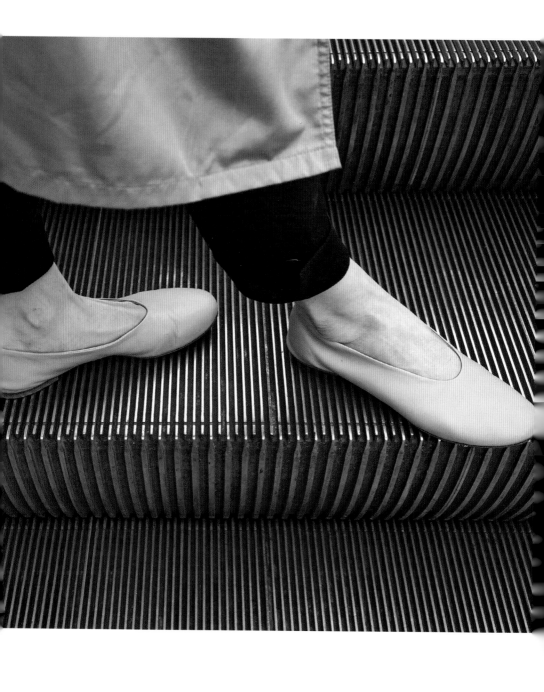

Take care of your feet

<hr>

It's hard to be mindful about your feet—until they start to hurt. And at that point, your feet become all you can think about. Body sustainability expert Yamuna Zake (known simply as Yamuna) says that almost every injury she sees in any part of the body comes back to the feet. If you set up a negative pattern from the feet, Yamuna explains, the problems just move up from there. Some people are helped by orthotics; others are not. But especially as we age, we can all benefit from regular daily foot care; it doesn't take a lot of time, and the relief can be huge. These suggestions are from Yamuna.

Switch up your shoes. Obviously, wearing high heels can be a problem, but even sneakers can cause trouble if you wear them all the time. Your feet need to walk in different shoes to stay nimble and healthy. So change it up. Have a range of comfortable shoes, and rotate them. And stop wearing any shoe that's causing pain. If shoes hurt, they're creating problems—not just during the time they're on your feet, but perhaps long-term.

Walk off the day barefoot. When you get home from work or running errands or exercising, take off your shoes as soon as you can and give your feet a chance to spread out. Walking barefoot engages all sorts of muscles that are squished and constricted most of the day. It's especially grounding to walk barefoot on a natural surface—grass, dirt, sand. Theoretically, a positive electromagnetic charge (which is a bad thing) builds up in our bodies from modern life—the food we eat, the stress we experience—and the negative electromagnetic charge emitted by the earth (which is good) can counteract that. But you need direct skin-to-earth contact to reap these theoretical benefits.

Roll out your feet. When possible, keep your feet moving and stimulated. If you have a desk job where you can discreetly pop off your shoes, keep a tennis ball or foot roller on the floor so you can massage soles while you work. It's the same principle as the foam roller, but in miniature. Yamuna sells smart simple tools to help with foot fitness at YamunaUSA.com and offers instruction online. She's a big believer in giving feet five or 10 minutes a day of stretching and range-of-motion activity. If you wear heels, at the very least stretch your feet, ankles, and calves at the end of the day: Standing with the ball of the foot on a step, allow your heel to drop as low as it wants to go. Stay and breathe, then switch sides.

Protect your skin

⸻⸻⸻⸻

Like your gut, your skin has a microbiome. What you put on it becomes part of that microbiome and also seeps into your bloodstream. So you want to choose carefully when it comes to soap, moisturizer, shampoo, and even perfume. Avoid chemicals in all self-care products. Here are some easy rules.

- **Use regular soap, not antibacterial.** First, a distinction: Hand sanitizer like Purell is an alcohol-based *disinfectant*—that's not the same as an antibacterial soap. Sanitizers that are 60 percent or more alcohol can kill a variety of germs and viruses on hands or surfaces. With concern about new viruses, hand sanitizer is a good backup. When you can't wash your hands with soap and water and you may have been exposed to something (say, after using a cart in the grocery store), use hand sanitizer. Antibacterial soap, which a lot of people buy reflexively for hand-washing at home, is something different. It's a chemical formulation that kills bacteria without distinguishing between the good bacteria your body needs and the bad bacteria it doesn't. There's less and less antibacterial soap on the market since a key ingredient (triclosan) was banned by the FDA, but it's still around. Don't use it. It won't help with a viral infection, and because it attacks the good bacteria in your body, it could hinder normal, healthy function of cells, tissues, and organs.

- **Beware bullsh*t beauty-product language.** There are many product lines with the veneer of purity that contain dangerous substances like sodium lauryl sulfate (SLS), sodium laureth sulfate (SLES), propylene glycol, petroleum, mineral oil (another name for petroleum), and chemical-y fragrance. Words like "plant-based," "natural," and "pure" are unregulated and meaningless. And just because a product is "paraben-free" doesn't mean it's not full of terrible ingredients. Read the actual label or, better yet, go to the Environmental Working Group's site (EWG.org) for details on safe skin-care and hair-care ingredients.

- **Take care of dryness.** Aging usually means drier skin, so in addition to good, pure moisturizer, gentle exfoliation is a good idea. A lot of people like dry-brushing before a shower. It feels good to sweep the skin clean and remove that dead layer. You don't need a lot of complicated products to restore moisture to the skin. Shop chemical-free brands like Drunk Elephant, Weleda, Dr. Hauschka, and Beautycounter. Or use organic creams and oils—shea butter, coconut oil, almond oil—straight up or blended. The book *Earthly Bodies & Heavenly Hair*, by clinical herbalist Dina Falconi, shares simple instructions for blending pure products using natural ingredients at home.

- **Defend the defender.** Don't overwash skin. The "acid mantle" is a microscopic layer that works as the skin's first line of defense against environmental pollutants and bacteria. You need this. So easy on the scrubbing, especially when it comes to your face; overcleansing destroys this natural, healthy barrier.

- **Keep an eye on sunspots, skin tags, and other unwelcome additions.** When things like this start appearing, an annual checkup by a dermatologist is a good idea. As with skin, some changes in hair, nails, and eyes come with aging and hormonal shifts. Everything will do better if you're getting the nutrients you need, not eating junk, and minimizing your intake of toxins in all ways, including through your pores.

Your mouth has a microbiome

Dental wellness is critical as you age. An imbalanced microbial colony in your mouth can hijack the immune system and create inflammation throughout the body. And many studies show that oral disease can lead to heart disease. Floss every day, and get your teeth cleaned twice a year. A burgeoning field of holistic dentistry (also called biological dentistry) looks at the oral microbiome in the greater context of the whole patient. It's like functional medicine for the mouth.

A book called *The Mouth-Body Connection*, by Dr. Gerry Curatola, is a good introduction to this type of thinking.

As with anything you put on or in your body, dental-care products should be as low in toxins as possible. Opt for natural toothpaste. Conventional toothpaste can contain concerning chemicals. A good brand called Revitin includes ingredients that support a healthy microbiome in the mouth; you can find it online.

Don't use Listerine or other antibacterial mouthwashes; these kill the good bacteria too. If breath is a problem, use a natural mouthwash, like Tom's of Maine. But bad breath is often a sign of some dysfunction in the gut—an imbalance in the microbiome—as is the state of the tongue. If there's a thick coating on your tongue or you have bad breath, what you really need to look at is your diet and the other things messing with your gut flora, like sleep and stress. Pay attention to problem foods. If, for example, dairy gives you a bellyache, it might also affect your breath; consider an elimination diet to ID the culprits. As you balance your gut microbiome and improve your diet—with fermented foods, lots of cruciferous vegetables, and especially stalks and stems—your breath should improve. As an alternative to mouthwash, some people like to swish with organic coconut oil, which is naturally antibacterial—this practice is called "oil pulling." It may be beneficial to the microbiome of the mouth.

And although age can bring with it less-white teeth (could be genetics, could be habits), you shouldn't whiten your teeth. Whitening products use bleach, which is a toxin you want to stay away from in all forms; they also contain hydrogen peroxide, which diffuses through the enamel and breaks down the compounds causing discoloration. But this can also irritate gums and damage dental enamel permanently. Instead, use charcoal toothpaste to whiten teeth. Charcoal, against all instincts, is a natural whitener that pulls stains from teeth. Burt's Bees makes a powdered version you can find at the drugstore; just brush it on, let it sit, then rinse well. Careful near the counter, sink, and towels, because it can stain. You can also find charcoal toothpaste in tubes, which is less messy.

Night eating means weight gain

Having a lot of food at night is the worst thing for your metabolism and for your sleep—and lack of sleep circles back and hurts metabolism. In terms of circadian rhythms, it's best to have most of your calories before 2 p.m. Your metabolism peaks around lunchtime, then begins to slow down; it doesn't break down calories as efficiently later in the day as it does midday. And at night? Well, many body functions are slowing as the "sleep function" prepares to take over. So if you eat then, you're more likely to store calories as fat than burn them as energy. Sumo wrestlers, when they're trying to put on weight, eat at night. It's a direct path to weight gain.

While plopping down in front of the TV with a snack is cozy, it interferes with optimal function. So even on days when you're not fasting for 16 hours, it's really important not to eat late at night—especially when you're stressed out. Here are answers to important questions about night eating.

What happens when you stress-eat at night?
The two hormones that get stimulated—cortisol, the stress hormone, and insulin, the blood-sugar hormone—are the perfect combination for gaining weight. When your cortisol level is high and your insulin level is high, this is the worst hormonal situation for weight gain and premature aging in general.

Is it true that it's hard to lose weight if you're not sleeping well? Why is that?
Yes, it's very hard to lose weight if you're not getting enough high-quality sleep. Lack of sleep increases the hormone ghrelin in the body, which causes you to feel hungry. At the same time, too little sleep leads to a lack of leptin, the hormone that makes you feel full. It's a double whammy.

What if I get home late and I'm starving, and I won't be able to fall asleep without something in my stomach?
Eat a handful of raw nuts or seeds, or have some avocado on flaxseed crackers. The point we're trying to make is that you should try to break the habit of snacking at night, not starve yourself if you missed dinner. In any case, don't eat too much, because it will keep you awake.

Is there anything I can have for fun while I'm watching TV?
Have a cup of tea—mint, chamomile, or something else without caffeine or other stimulants. When you experience how much more easily you sleep without that late-night snack, you might not find it so hard to give up. Over time, brewing and drinking tea can become that relaxing ritual that your body craves, in place of snacking.

Find comrades in aging well

It can be tricky to improve your habits and stick with a new lifestyle if your partner isn't on the same path. We're not looking to blame anyone—your health journey is your own responsibility—but altering diet, exercise, and everyday practices toward best-case aging is easier with a coconspirator. Ideally, that's the person you live with. Because if not, it's hard. Junk food in the cupboard, a bright TV blaring at bedtime, texts pinging at all hours, a resistance to getting up and out of the house—these can become serious stressors and can strain a relationship.

One idea for drawing in your partner is to suggest one small change you can easily do together as a couple, like intermittent fasting. It's not too challenging (like a lifestyle overhaul might be), but it can be really bonding. We see many people who notice an immediate difference, and become inspired.

That personal, subjective sensation of feeling better, for many folks, turns into commitment. Or you could agree to drop one thing from your cupboards or fridge (say, sugar!). Embarking on a tiny doable wellness adventure together can be very positive, and might lead to a shared effort to improve other elements.

If this kind of thing isn't on the table, find a pal who's enthusiastic about wellness. We know it's not a small thing if your life partner isn't with you on this. It not only feels lonely but can also be painful and upsetting—you worry about the people you love and want the best for them, and if your partner isn't taking great care of themself, that can mean ongoing tension. But don't let this get in the way. Take care of yourself. Maybe some of your good habits will rub off. Aging well is not a one-step proposition. It can be a slow build of practices—one habit replacing another. Put on your own oxygen mask, and be sure you have a buddy who's thinking like you are. Having company makes it easier to stick with new practices.

Snacking strategies

In a perfect world, there are organic carrot sticks, guacamole, and raw walnuts at your fingertips at all times. But here on earth, you have to plan for different scenarios. Start by rethinking what qualifies as a snack. Protein bars should not be a regular part of your snacking life. Most of the popular brands are full of sugar. Here are some great snacking ideas from health coach Dawn Brighid.

- A cup of bone broth
- Tea (or coffee) with a scoop of collagen and cashew milk
- A sliced green apple with unsweetened almond butter
- Half an avocado with olive oil and sea salt
- A handful of nuts or seeds
- A half cup of olives
- Dairy-free pesto with veggies or flaxseed crackers
- Grass-fed and organic beef, turkey, or salmon jerky (see WildZora.com for some great options)

Desperate circumstances can make it tough to stay on the low-carb wagon, so have policies in place for worst-case food situations—working late, starving at the airport, road trips. Raw nuts are a great go-to (better than, say, a banana, which is high in sugar), and you can find them just about everywhere. Why not roasted nuts? Because roasting generally involves problematic oil (dry-roasted is fine). Decent protein bars are those that are low in sugar, like Dang Bars, Love Good Fats Bars, Bulletproof Bars, IQ Bars, and Health Warrior Chia Bars. But don't make a habit of them. Instead, if you crave a sweet, have a few squares of dark chocolate. It should have a high cocoa concentration (80 percent or higher) and very little sugar (no more than 4 grams per serving).

Gardening for aging well

In Scotland, doctors can now prescribe time in nature to reduce blood pressure and anxiety for those with diabetes, stress, heart disease, and more. Here in the United States, we're absurdly slow to catch up, but we don't need to wait till the AMA gets it. Trees, dirt, sunshine, sand, water—these are good for you. You know how cleansed and refreshed you feel when you sit on a beach with the wind blowing in your hair. You know the peace of walking on soft rich ground in the forest. You can feel that something is happening when you let the sun shine on your face. We are solar-powered. And nature, in any form, is healing, soothing, energizing.

For many of us, the easiest way to commune with nature is through gardening and other yard work. Digging in the dirt, absorbing sunshine, inhaling fresh air, squatting, reaching and pulling, using your hands and body in a way that's different and varied, being outside—it's like a complete protein of physical and psychological wellness. Functional movement meets fresh air meets exposure to microbes in the soil meets beauty. It's the composite activity of everything in this book—a fast path to multiple benefits. If you don't have a garden, look into community gardens. Offer to help out a neighbor who may not have the time or agility to keep up with their garden. Search for local volunteer opportunities to get your hands dirty in this joyous way.

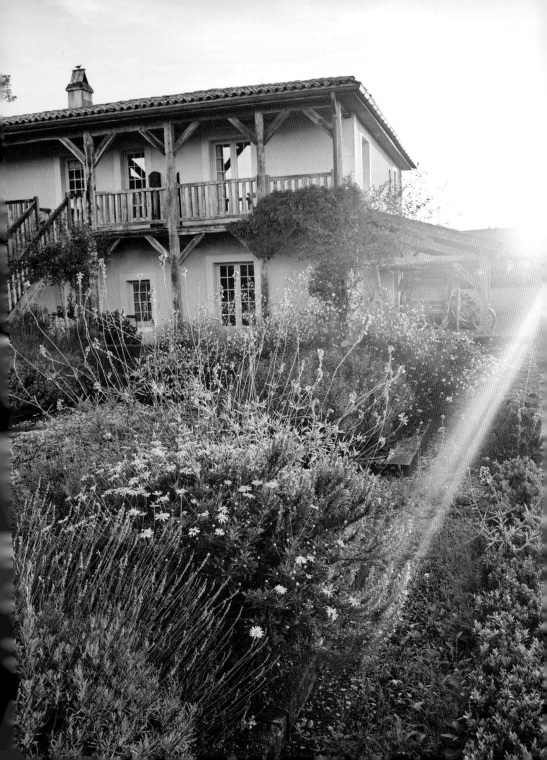

Timing your wellness life

Aging well is not about perfection; it's about consistency. Here's a snapshot of great practices in context, to show how organic (and easy) it can be to integrate new habits.

MORNING

- Stretch in bed.
- Step outside first thing if possible. Sunshine on your face helps keep your circadian rhythms in a good place and connects you with nature, which will help your sleep later on.

- Switch your hot shower to cold for the last 30 seconds.
- Meditate or do some conscious breathing at home or on your commute, if possible.
- Have a cup of coffee or tea with MCT oil for a big energy boost.

DAYTIME

- Move around at work as much as possible, and use break time for a walk uphill or up stairs.
- Keep some supplements at work or in your bag in case you forget to take them at home.
- Fill up on fiber and fat—a green salad and a handful of nuts, for example—at midday to get ahead of that looming afternoon energy drop.

- Drink a glass of filtered water whenever you take a break from your work.
- Grab a few minutes in the sun with a friend.
- Do errands on foot, and take the longer, hillier route.

EVENING

- Take off your shoes when you get home, and go barefoot.
- Relax after work with your legs up on the wall.
- Have dinner on the early side so you can begin your food break/overnight fast without stressing (aim to finish eating three hours before bed).
- Put away leftovers and do the dishes right after dinner, so you're not tempted to snack as you clean later. (Think of the kitchen as closed after cleanup.)
- Turn off screens and set devices to charge away from the bedroom.
- Lower the temperature of your bedroom.

NIGHT

- Sit down with a cup of chamomile or mint tea to help close out the eating part of your day and begin your wind-down.
- Take your magnesium supplement.
- Take a bath or relax in a restorative yoga pose.
- If you haven't been getting enough sleep, get in bed an hour earlier than usual (and if you have to choose between morning exercise and high-quality sleep, choose sleep).
- Read a book on paper, not on-screen. Wait till your eyes are really heavy, then turn out the light.

INNER HEALTH

———

Cultivating joy, happiness, calm,
intimacy, and curiosity: Don't ignore these soft
(but crucial) aspects of aging well.

Take in good things

Your diet isn't just what you eat but whom you hang out with, what you listen to, what you read, where you spend your free time, what you watch on-screen. It's everything you take in.

Do you find it impossible to look away from the stressful 24-hour news cycle? Are there negative people in your life who routinely leave you feeling terrible? Does social media eat up whole chunks of your night? Is gossip a big part of your life?

Step back and take inventory. Maybe you can "unsubscribe" from some of the things that cause you agita: news sources, human beings, activities. Look out for social situations—even casual small-talky moments—that are toxic. Get away from complainers; they sap your strength. Instead, make it a point to spend time with can-do, positive people who inspire and motivate you. Read books and articles that enrich you and feed curiosity to balance the negatives of the news. Pour in the good stuff. It helps you cultivate the best parts of yourself, and stay positive as you age, which can have a profound impact on your health.

While you're at it, make a point of practicing active kindness. Tip your server well, return your shopping cart, let someone into your lane on the highway, hold the door. Look for opportunities to be of service. Live positively. This helps

(continues on page 210)

People need people

"**Rosemary, 61,** comes in and tells me she's feeling foggy. She can't focus and has trouble staying on task. She's putting on weight, feeling fatigued, not getting decent sleep. Rosemary recently lost her husband. Her kids live far away.

She's always loved gardening but now is feeling too tired to do it. Her blood tests show a mildly sluggish thyroid and a very low level of pregnenolone. Pregnenolone is a hormone naturally produced by the adrenal glands. It's also the starting material for the production of many of our other hormones, including cortisol, progesterone, estrogen, and testosterone.

In talking with Rosemary, I discover that she's isolated. Without her husband, who was her constant companion, she's home alone most of the time. Her friends dropped by a lot at first and now invite her out occasionally, but she feels too tired to go and usually declines. She's ordinarily a physical, athletic person but has been unmotivated to bike or go to the gym.

I suggest Rosemary start taking a restorative yoga class. This is a low-stress way to move her body and be around more people. Loneliness can be as bad for you as any chronic disease. I give her adaptogens and nutrients for adrenal and thyroid support. We keep the bar low—the only changes I ask her to make are to go to yoga and to make a small effort to prepare better for sleep every night.

We meet again two weeks later. Rosemary is sleeping better; she's feeling less down and more alert. She's lost a little bit of weight. We talk about what's going on. Now that she's feeling a bit better, I tell her to get some more people in her life, start looking intentionally for new tribes she might belong with. Social support is crucial.

It takes a while, but six months later when I next see Rosemary, she's joined a group for environmentally conscious people who want to grow their own food. They meet biweekly and help in each other's vegetable gardens. Her energy is up, and she's booked a bike trip in the Southwest with an old friend. She trains every day. She's started to look forward, and her conversation is peppered with the word 'we,' which is a positive sign. She's finding her people, and her health shows it."

THINK ABOUT IT:

- How big is your social circle? Do you want to expand it?

- What's your favorite way to see friends, one-on-one or in a group? Doing something active or sitting and talking?

- What would be a fun weekly social activity?

- What do you look forward to, short term and long term?

- What gets you out of the house, and will keep getting you out of the house?

- Who are the people you depend on?

- Have you ever had your hormone levels checked?

- What's one tiny change you can make today toward more activity or joy?

you develop a lightness about life and all its imperfections. Cultivate patience. If a friend is late, can you enjoy looking at the trees? If the driver in front of you doesn't step on the gas the moment the light turns green, can you cut them some slack? Think of the oft-memed Ian Maclaren quote: "Be kind. For everyone you meet is fighting a battle you know nothing about."

You have the choice in every situation to pursue compassion. It's an excellent way to age. It will help you get and stay happy, and it will draw others to you.

Relax like a cat, play like a dog

You probably don't need a book to tell you that loving and caring for an animal is good for your health. But studies show that people who have pets live longer, happier, healthier lives. Anyone who's a pet parent can attest to the myriad ways cats and dogs enrich life. Shelters are full of sweet cats and dogs that need homes; many are older, trained, and mellow. If you don't have a pet, now is a great time to consider adopting.

Cats and dogs have lessons to teach us about aging well— they're constant reminders of how to live simply and better: stretching out in the sun, resting when you're tired, cuddling up in bed with someone you love. Using your senses to take in and appreciate the world around you. Frolicking in the surf,

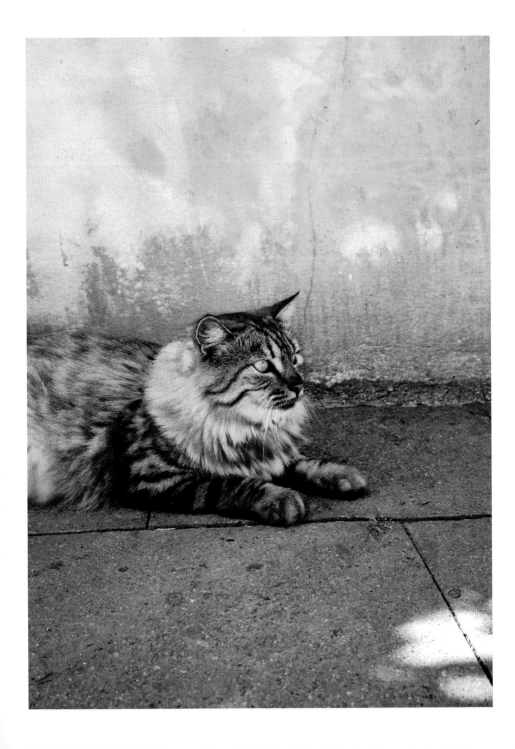

catching balls, running out and back for no reason. Being curious, being present, enjoying food and walks and company. Whether you're a cat person or a dog person, having a creature to care for is more a gift to you than anything else—and one of the secrets to ongoing vitality.

Dogs in particular keep you youthful by getting you out of the house every single morning. Walking a dog also tends to bring with it incidental socializing—you chat with folks at the dog park, and stop on the street for those who want to meet your pet. These little interactions are emotional vitamins, and as we age, they're more and more important. If you're thinking of adopting, go for it.

Let go of grudges

Nelson Mandela said, "Resentment is like drinking poison and then hoping it will kill your enemies."

What are you carrying that you can drop? It's human nature to, at times, become imprisoned by resentments. But if you can let go of anger, forgive the person you're mad at, move on from a grudge, it will help your physical health.

If there's something that needs to be discussed, talk about it. If there's an issue you need to work through on your own, go to therapy or confront it with the help of another practice. Meditation, philosophy, somatic healing, religion, past-life regression, breathwork—whatever speaks to you. Do it. Go there. Move through it.

You may not have the power to get justice, to garner an apology, to gain real closure, but you do have the power to let go. Even if you're completely right, even if you can't get the resolution you crave, holding on to anger punishes no one more than you. Over months and years and decades, it can have negative effects on your health. Sit for a moment with the feeling of a grudge—ignore the storyline and just see what you feel in your body. It might manifest as tightness in a specific body part, or as held breath, or as an overall clenched sensation. This is what we want to relieve you of. Put your health first, and let it go.

Carve new pathways

As life shifts and time opens up, filling the space with activities you love is key to staying vital. Don't wait till later. Weave in new elements now—seed the ground. Take a class, revive a hobby, find something that gets you going.

Download that language-learning app. Dust off the guitar. Learn to code or tango or forage in the woods. Cultivate personal, self-propelled, dependable joy.

Maybe what moves you is helping others. Don't put it off for some distant future. Volunteer now. Think about what

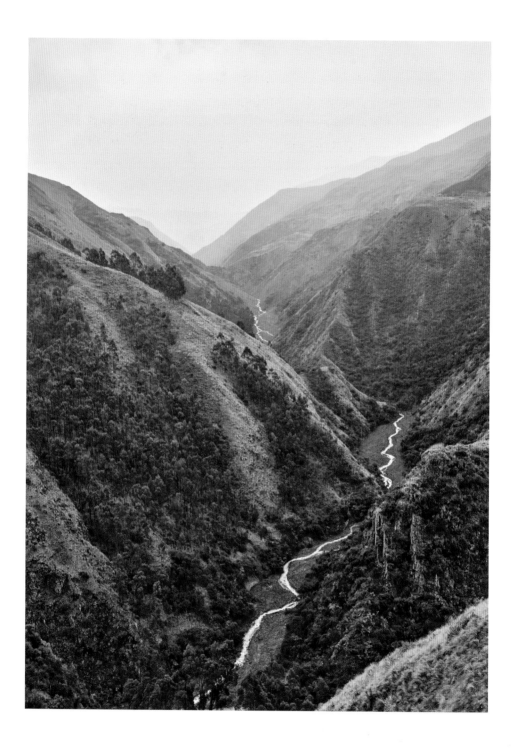

gifts you have to offer (cooking, reading, teaching, driving) and whom you like to help (animals, kids, older humans). If you pick well and start with a small commitment, volunteering will feel more like a gift than a chore. Find out about drop-in days at an animal shelter, cleanup efforts at a local park, meal-prep groups for homebound folks. What you get back is invaluable, and becoming involved with like-minded people expands your community.

Go forward with an attitude of "why not?" Let an ethos of moving and growing inform your world. Whatever you've got tucked away in your "someday" file, tap into it as soon as you can. Travel, adventure, creative pursuits, giving of yourself—it's all about looking out and up. And it's a great way to prep for upcoming chapters of life while enriching the one you're in.

AFTERWORD

Many of the core practices in this book have been known in different cultures for centuries. We didn't make up this stuff or even discover it, but we're glad to be able to help people get back to it. Walking in nature, having quiet time, moving the body, eating what grows near us, being an active part of a community—this is ageless wisdom. We want to acknowledge and thank ancient medicine for its common-sense brilliance and offer a nod to modern science for rekindling respect for the simple intuitive practices of healthy aging.

GREAT RESOURCES

The Blue Zones: Nine Lessons for Living Longer from the People Who've Lived the Longest, by Dan Buettner

The Complete Guide to Fasting: Heal Your Body Through Intermittent, Alternate-Day, and Extended Fasting, by Jason Fung, MD, and Jimmy Moore

The End of Alzheimer's: The First Program to Prevent and Reverse Cognitive Decline, by Dale E. Bredesen, MD

Grain Brain: The Surprising Truth about Wheat, Carbs, and Sugar— Your Brain's Silent Killers, by David Perlmutter, MD, and Kristin Loberg

I Contain Multitudes: The Microbes Within Us and a Grander View of Life, by Ed Yong

Lifespan: Why We Age—and Why We Don't Have To, by David A. Sinclair, PhD

The Mouth-Body Connection, by Dr. Gerry Curatola

Practical Wisdom: The Right Way to Do the Right Thing, by Barry Schwartz and Kenneth Sharpe

The Rebel's Apothecary: A Practical Guide to the Healing Magic of Cannabis, CBD, and Mushrooms, by Jenny Sansouci

Six Seasons: A New Way with Vegetables, by Joshua McFadden and Martha Holmberg

ACKNOWLEDGMENTS

Thank you to my coauthor, Danielle Claro; all the folks at Artisan Books; and my longtime agent, Stephanie Tade. Thank you to my staff and colleagues at the Eleven Eleven Wellness Center, who have supported me for so many years and helped create a new model of health care. Thank you to the staff and my colleagues at The Well, who have created a special place and a burgeoning, progressive wellness community. Thank you to my patients, who continually teach me and inspire me to explore new ways for all of us to become and stay healthier. Thank you to my daughter and son-in-law, Alison and Zach, who challenge me to keep it real. And finally, thank you to my beautiful wife, Janice, who for more than 40 years has been there for me in every way possible. I could not do any of this without her. I dedicate this book to our new grandson, Benjamin, who has given me even more reasons to age well and stay vital for another 40 years. —F. L.

Deep thanks to our publisher, Lia Ronnen; our editor, Shoshana Gutmajer; and the entire hardworking team at Artisan Books, including Suet Chong, Jane Treuhaft, Sibylle Kazeroid, Annie O'Donnell, and Nancy Murray. Gratitude to my coauthor, Frank Lipman, whom I quote in conversation more often than any other human except Tina Fey. Thank you to Gentl and Hyers for the beautiful photos in this book— a spoonful of raspberries to help the health advice go down. Thanks to my close people: Beth Kobliner, Liz Kiernan, Wendy

Odabashian, Pascale Le Draoulec, and especially Jeff Eyrich, who has aged backward in the time I've known him. Thank you to my folks, Fran and Joe Claro, for their inspiration and their good Italian genes. Thanks to my kids, Ian Reilly and Ruby Reilly, and my daughter's partner, KT Firstenberger, for their unfailing love and support. Thanks to Alan Stein, Renata Di Biase, Mary Ford-Sussman, Mary-Ann Mastreani, Naomi Ortiz, Dina Falconi, and the wonderful teachers at Now Yoga for boosting my own joy and wellness quotient. Thanks to Muddy Water Café, my office away from home, HudCo work space, and Elsa Ordahl for her organizational help. And thanks to the friends and neighbors who stopped me at the farmers' market and around town with specific questions on aging well: Your curiosity about everything from turmeric to tequila helped shape this book. —D. C.

INDEX

"Be kind whenever possible.
It is always possible."

—*the Dalai Lama*